Nursing: Decision-Making Skills for Practice

Edited by **Karen Holland** and **Deborah Roberts**

Series editor **Karen Holland**

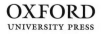

OXFORD
UNIVERSITY PRESS

OXFORD
UNIVERSITY PRESS

Great Clarendon Street, Oxford, OX2 6DP,
United Kingdom

Oxford University Press is a department of the University of Oxford.
It furthers the University's objective of excellence in research, scholarship,
and education by publishing worldwide. Oxford is a registered trade mark of
Oxford University Press in the UK and in certain other countries

British Library Cataloguing in Publication Data
Data available

ISBN 978-0-19-964142-0

Printed in Great Britain by
Ashford Colour Press Ltd, Gosport, Hampshire

Oxford University Press makes no representation, express or implied, that
the drug dosages in this book are correct. Readers must therefore always check
the product information and clinical procedures with the most up-to-date
published product information and data sheets provided by the manufacturers
and the most recent codes of conduct and safety regulations. The authors and
the publishers do not accept responsibility or legal liability for any errors in the
text or for the misuse or misapplication of material in this work. Except where
otherwise stated, drug dosages and recommendations are for the non-pregnant
adult who is not breast-feeding.

Links to third party websites are provided by Oxford in good faith and for information only.
Oxford disclaims any responsibility for the materials contained in any third party website
referenced in this work.

Series editor preface

Learning to be a nurse requires students to develop a set of skills and a knowledge base which will enable them to make the transition from learner to qualified nurse. As with any transition this can often seem at times to be a daunting prospect, and one where the student may ask 'how am I ever going to learn all that I need to know to get through this course and become a qualified nurse?'

For student nurses this experience entails learning in 'two worlds', that of the university and that of the clinical environment. Although there is a physical distinction between the two, it is important that the learning that takes place in one is integrated with the learning in the other. This series of books has set out to do just that.

These 'two worlds' require that students learn two sets of skills in order to qualify as a nurse and be ready to take on further sets of skills in whatever nursing environment they are employed. The skills which will be a core part of this series are numerous, and central to them is that of 'coping with the unknown'. This being in relation to facing a new environment each time they start a new clinical placement, communicating with patients and a large number of health and social care professionals, dealing with difficult and often complex situations and sometimes stressful clinical experiences. In the university there are also situations which may be unknown, such as learning new study skills, working with others, searching and finding information, and managing workloads. It is every student's goal to complete their course with the required foundation for the future and it is the essential goal of this series to enable the student to develop skills for a successful learning and nursing experience.

The central ethos to all the books therefore is to facilitate and enhance the student learning experience and develop their skills, through engaging with a variety of reflective accounts, exercises and web-based resources. We hope that you as the reader and learner enjoy reading these books and that the guidance within them supports your goal of successfully completing your course of study.

Karen Holland
Series Editor

Preface

Decision making is a critical element of day-to-day practice for any nurse working in a health care environment. Decisions can be related to clinical care, ranging from helping a patient to decide what to eat (to ensure the balanced nutritional intake essential for well-being) or deciding how best to feed the patient who has had a stroke, to more complex decisions such as those required to resuscitate someone who has had a heart attack. Central to all such decision making is involving the patients/clients and, where appropriate, their carers.

Nursing decisions can also involve deciding how to prioritize workloads, deciding what evidence to use for a care plan, or deciding if you are competent to undertake a certain task. These may not directly involve the patient in the decision-making process, but will fundamentally affect either the evidence-based care developed or the way in which care is delivered.

To engage in effective decision making, the student requires a set of skills, underpinned by the most appropriate knowledge and best evidence, which they need to acquire during the course of their learning to become a nurse. In its new 2010 Standards, the Nursing and Midwifery Council (NMC) now recognizes the importance of decision-making skills as a specific area of competence necessary when registering as a nurse.

Our aim in this book is to facilitate the learning experience of the student by providing him or her with an insight into real-world examples of decision making in action, supported by a foundation of knowledge that he or she will be required to use in his or her own experience, and which is also fundamental to achieving the key competencies of the NMC Standards (2010). It is anticipated that the book will support student learning throughout the course, and will meet students' needs with regards to the foundation skills and knowledge required for effective decision making in all fields of practice.

Contents

About the editors

Karen Holland

Karen is Editor-in-Chief of the international Nurse Education in Practice journal. She is author of six published books (one translated into Japanese). She is currently Series Editor of a series of books for Oxford University Press and another publisher. She has a specific research interest in student learning in practice, partnership working, practice development and curriculum innovations and has undertaken and led a number of research projects and development work in these fields. She is totally committed to ensuring the quality of the student learning experience and to ensuring that nursing education has a rigorous evidence- base. She is a member of the international Content Selection & Advisory Board (CSAB) for SCOPUS (Elsevier) where she is one of the 14 Subject Chairs (Nursing/Health Professions/Education). This role involves evaluation of all journals submitted to the subject fields for inclusion in the SCOPUS database.

Deborah Roberts

Dr Deborah Roberts is a Reader in Nursing at Glyndwr University, Wales and has been a nurse lecturer since 2000, following 13 years in clinical practice. Deborah has published widely on issues related to teaching and learning in nurse education and regularly presents at conferences. Her PhD research concerned peer learning: how and where student nurses learn from each other.

About the contributors

Deborah Atkinson   Director of Nursing, Mastercall Healthcare

Ruth Chadwick   Senior Lecturer and Student Facing Processes Lead, School of Nursing, Midwifery and Social Work, University of Salford

Joanne Cleary-Holdforth   Lecturer in Nursing, School of Nursing and Human Sciences, Dublin City University

Dawn Gawthorpe   Senior Lecturer, School of Nursing, Midwifery and Social Work, University of Salford

Sue Hart   Nurse Coordinator for NHS Surrey and Freelance Trainer

Gareth Holland   Staff nurse, Adult Forensic Unit, North West of England

June Keeling   Senior Lecturer, Faculty of Health and Social Care, University of Chester

Mike Lappin   Lecturer in Adult Nursing, School of Nursing, Midwifery and Social Work, University of Salford

Thérèse Leufer   Lecturer in Nursing, School of Nursing and Human Sciences, Dublin City University

Aatefa Lunat   Neonatal Staff Nurse, Neonatal Unit, North West of England

Denise Major   Lecturer, Children's and Young People's Nursing, University of Salford

Jane McGrath   (Newly qualified) Staff Nurse, Acute Medical Unit (AMU), North West England

Sarah Ratcliffe   Lecturer in Adult Nursing, School of Nursing, Midwifery and Social Work, University of Salford

Eva Scarlett   Learning Disabilities Nurse, South of England

Joyce Smith   Lecturer in Adult Nursing, School of Nursing, Midwifery and Social Work, University of Salford

Jenni Templeman   Senior Lecturer and Deputy Programme Lead, University of Chester

Tony Warne   Professor in Mental Health Care, School of Nursing, Midwifery and Social Work, University of Salford

How to use this book

Nursing: Decision-Making Skills for Practice outlines the skills that students and nurses need to make effective and safe decisions. This brief tour of the book shows readers how to get the most out of this textbook.

Finding your way through

Find what you need fast The list of contents in the front of the book and the list of learning objectives at the beginning of each chapter will help you navigate this book.

Bringing theory to life

Numbered boxes highlight extra information to help you take your understanding further.

Exercises and Activities help you to test your knowledge and put theory into real-world situations.

Case studies present you with situations you're likely to encounter as a qualified nurse and help you plan how you might react.

Reflection points give you a chance to reflect on situations you've experienced in the past, and how you might learn from them to improve your practice.

Next steps

Summaries at the end of every chapter conclude what has been covered and give you the opportunity to assess your progress.

Further reading lists direct you to the best sources of evidence and information for more in-depth study.

PART 1

Decision making:
theory and practice

PART 1

This part of the book will focus on the theoretical and evidence base underpinning decision making for nursing. It is important that you are able to understand the rationale for making different kinds of decisions, as well as ensure that, whenever possible, your decisions are underpinned by an evidence base. Being able to understand the evidence for your decisions is not enough, however, to change or develop further your decision-making skills, which is why there is a focus on reflection and reflective practice in the book. Reflecting on your experiences in a structured way can help you to identify a different way of making similar decisions or, alternatively, it can help you to use that experience and to apply the learning to a range of other decisions.

Principles of decision making

Karen Holland and Deborah Roberts

The aims of this chapter are to:

- ➜ outline the principles of decision making as they affect the role of the student nurse;
- ➜ consider why learning to make decisions is an important part of learning to become a nurse;
- ➜ consider the skills and knowledge necessary for effective decision making in both clinical and university learning settings; and
- ➜ consider what is known about decision making as a student nurse.

Introduction

The focus of this book is decision-making skills for practice and, as such, it will become apparent not only that it is essential for student nurses to learn about what these skills are, but also that it is equally important that they learn to become competent in making the decisions that are an essential part of becoming a qualified nurse.

As individuals, we make decisions of one form or another on a daily basis. We have to make basic decisions such as what time to get up in the morning, what to wear that day, who is going to take the children to school, or what to have for breakfast. These decisions do not appear, on their surface, to require major consideration when it comes to decision making, but for some people even these seemingly basic decision-making situations can cause immense stress, resulting either from the act of decision making itself or from having to take into account the context, or impact on others, of any decision taken. Some of you will come across patients or clients in whom this has developed into a health-related problem and we will be considering these issues in later chapters. Your ability to become a confident decision maker in practice will, however, be dependent on the decisions that you make as a student in the university and as a person. Some of the situations in which making decisions impacts on all aspects of your learning to become a nurse will be discussed in **Chapter 2**.

This chapter is initially concerned with the underlying principles of decision making as a student nurse. It explores why it is important and necessary to learn about decision making, and how to make decisions; it will also focus on what has been shown in the literature about decision making as both a student nurse and a qualified nurse, and most importantly what you need to achieve to meet the Nursing and Midwifery Council (NMC) competencies. Later chapters will focus on the application of some of this learning to specific practice contexts and situations.

So where to begin? For students studying in the United Kingdom, we begin with the NMC's *Standards for Pre-Registration Nursing Education* (NMC 2010). Those of you studying in other countries can use the competencies outlined in this book as a guide and consider some of your own country-specific professional body requirements on decision-making skills alongside those that apply in the UK. Because nursing is a global profession, however, regardless of in which country you are learning to become a nurse, it may be of use to you to access the relevant standards or competencies required to see what the expectations are of a qualified nurse in each country. Given the way in which qualified nurses cross international borders to work, this will give you an added insight into what may be expected of you should you choose to work in another country on qualifying.

The requirements of the Nursing and Midwifery Council Standards (2010)

In view of the importance of decision making to both your learning as a student and your need to achieve those NMC (2010) competencies that involve decision making, it may be relevant to begin with the latter: meeting the NMC competencies. At the present time, there are two different sets of NMC Standards: those published in 2004 and those published in 2010, the latter being compulsory for all students commencing the graduate-only programmes in the UK starting September 2013 (NMC 2010), when nursing becomes an all-graduate profession. It is these more recent Standards to which we will mainly be referring in this book, but recognizing the importance also of helping all students undergoing a programme of learning to becoming a qualified nurse and who will have to meet a similar set of competencies for registration as a nurse on the NMC register.

The NMC Standards (2010) comprise four main 'domains', each of which requires the student nurse to be able to learn how to make decisions that are underpinned by an evidence base and a clear decision-making pathway. These domains cover the following areas.

1. Professional values
2. Communication and interpersonal skills

3. Nursing practice and decision making
4. Leadership, management, and team working

Each one of these domains has a generic standard of competence (which applies to all student nurses regardless of their intended field of practice), a field standard of competence, and a number of specific generic and field-specific competencies, all of which are expected to be achieved by the end of the student's programme of learning in both practice placement and university assessments.

To be able to make decisions applicable to these four domains, you will need to understand the various principles underpinning the variety of decisions that you will be required to make as a student nurse learning to become a qualified nurse, as well as to know why they are appropriate for certain decisions and not for others. **Part 1** of this book, comprising this chapter and three others, is intended to give you this theoretical foundation.

We will then focus in **Part 2** on possible generic decisions and decision making that you may have to make in relation to each of the four domains themselves. In **Part 3**, we build on this knowledge to focus on the field-specific decisions that you may come across in each of the four fields of practice: mental health nursing; children and young people's nursing; adult nursing; and learning disability nursing. Although these chapters focus on field-specific issues relevant to those of you following one of the four field-specific pathways, the content is applicable to any student learning to make nursing decisions, in keeping with the need to engage in what is known as 'exposure to other fields of practice'—a requirement of the NMC Standards.

Activity

1. Visit <http://standards.nmc-uk.org/PreRegNursing/statutory/competencies/Pages/Competencies.aspx> and familiarize yourselves with the domains, generic competencies, and field-specific competencies relevant to your field-of-practice pathway to registration. (For some of you reading this book, this refers to your Branch and to decision making in the context of the NMC 2004 Standards.)

2. Identify those 'Progression criteria' (Annexe 2 to the Standards) that you are required to achieve at the end of the year in which you are currently, such as the 'First progression point criteria', which you are expected to have achieved by the end of Year 1, of which Table 1.1 is one criterion.

3. Consider what decisions in relation to this competence you will be expected to demonstrate as a student nurse, what knowledge you will be expected to have on which to base the decisions, and against what criteria your mentor will be assessing whether you have achieved that competence.

Table 1.1 Example of first progression point criteria (NMC Standards 2010)

Areas associated with safety and safeguarding people of all ages, their carers and their families	Related competency domains
...	...
4. Is able to recognize when a person's physical or psychological condition is deteriorating, demonstrating how to act in an emergency and administer essential first aid.	Nursing practice and decision making Leadership, management and team working

Source: <http://standards.nmc-uk.org/Documents/Annexe2_progression_criteria_20100916.pdf>

The principles of decision making and their relevance to learning to become a qualified nurse

If you are expected to achieve the NMC competencies, many of which require decision making of one sort or another, then it is important to consider the different types of decision making that you can make, as well as the theoretical principles underpinning them. You will note references to these throughout the book. In addition, you will find many articles and books that refer to the use of 'clinical decision making'—that is, decision making in those situations that require a decision based on either a set of *clinical data* related to a patient, which can be analysed to make a 'clinical' decision, such as giving pain relief following assessment of patient needs, and a set of *cues* from the patient, which indicates that he or she is in pain, or alternatively on the *best evidence from research*, which can be used to change clinical practice decisions, such as what type of pain relief can be given to the patient in pain. All of these are 'clinical' in the sense that they are decisions made with regards to direct patient care.

One could argue that any decision that takes place in the clinical environment that has a direct or indirect impact on patient care could be considered to be an example of clinical decision making. We will see, however, that students have to make a wide variety of other decisions relevant to their learning to become nurses, including basic decisions such as attending a lecture. Regardless of the type of decision making, there will always be a possible positive or negative outcome to that decision, which will depend on the information available on which to base the decision. In **Chapter 2**, we look at a broad range of decision-making opportunities and options with which you will be faced as a student nurse studying for a degree in nursing, combined with registration as a qualified nurse. **Chapter 3** focuses on how we gather and use evidence in the decision-making process, an understanding of which is an essential prerequisite to becoming a registered nurse. In **Chapter 4**, we will look at the set of tools that you can use to help in the decision-making process; we focus on one of these in particular—that is, reflection and decision making—which appears to be a central core of most students' curriculum.

So how do you learn to make decisions and what underpins the decision-making process that you undertake?

Decision-making theories: the basics

Here, we intend to introduce you to the basics of decision making so that you can consider how decisions are made in practice—but it is important to remember that you need to undertake further reading at various stages of your course of learning. (See the '**Further reading**' at the end of chapter for some examples.)

The three main decision-making theories are, according to Aston et al. (2010: 7):

- the information-processing model;
- the intuition model; and
- the cognitive continuum theory.

Although other authors, such as Thompson and Dowding (2009), and Standing (2010), expand on these three models, the basic principles remain the same. They are mainly used in the context of clinical decision making rather than more general principles of decision making. You may, however, come across terms such as 'hypothetico-deductive reasoning' (Thompson and Dowding 2009: 63), which follows several 'different stages of reasoning when making judgements and decisions', consisting in essence of four basic stages:

1. 'cue acquisition' (collecting clinical information);
2. 'hypothesis generation' (at which point possible options might be considered based on the data gathered);
3. 'cue interpretation' (the point at which the data is examined closer and, together with the 'whole picture', used to consider a revised decision or possibility); and
4. 'cue evaluation' (the point at which you might decide that, despite having an idea about what you need to do or what the problem could be, a rethink is needed and perhaps some more data is required, or even that you need to repeat your data collection, to check its accuracy).

After following these stages, you will be able to make a more definite decision based on the best possible clinical data.

Jones (1996) outlines an important relationship between other skills that are required in relation to the decision-making process, such as 'critical thinking' and 'critical analysis' (Tappen 1989). These, she defines as follows:

Critical thinking is a skill developed in looking for alternative solutions to problems and adopting a questioning approach. *Critical analysis* is a tool used in critical thinking and may involve asking the following questions:

- *What is the central issue?*
- *What are the underlying assumptions?*

- Is there valid evidence?
- Are the conclusions acceptable?

  These questions help analyse the steps in the decision-making process.

  (Jones 1996: 3)

Both critical thinking and critical analysis are key concepts throughout the book, and examples of situations in which these are used by students and their mentors in practice will be explored, as well as examples of their use in academic learning in the university. Both are skills that can be taught and learned, and are considered essential for the graduate qualified nurse of the future; along with decision-making skills, they underpin the clinical and managerial leadership roles that will be expected of that nurse.

Two additional terms associated with decision making in practice are 'clinical reasoning' and 'clinical judgement'. We will define them briefly here, to help to identify the links between them and the decision-making process, but we return to these later in the chapter.

- **Clinical reasoning** is defined by Levett-Jones et al. (2010: 516) as:

a logical process by which nurses (and other clinicians) collect cues, process the information, come to an understanding of a patient problem or situation, plan and implement interventions, evaluate outcomes and reflect in and learn from the process (Hoffman 2007). It is not a linear process but can be conceptualized as a cycle of linked clinical encounters.

- **Clinical judgement**, according to Benner et al. (1996: 2), refers to

'*the ways in which nurses come to understand the problems, issues or concerns of clients/patients, to attend to salient information, and to respond in concerned and involved ways*'.

Tanner (2006) subsequently developed a clinical judgement model that consists of four phases—*noticing, interpreting, responding,* and *reflecting*—which Lasater (2007: 497) describes as

'*the major components of clinical judgement in complex patient care situations that involve changes in status and uncertainty about the appropriate course of action*'.

Tanner (2006: 204) concluded in her research that

'*reflection on practice is often triggered by a breakdown in clinical judgement and is critical for the development of clinical knowledge and improvement in clinical reasoning*'.

This concept of 'reflection' in the decision-making process, and its use and experience, are discussed in more detail in **Chapter 4**.

In addition to these decision-making processes and problem-solving tools, there are other frameworks that we can use to determine when certain types of decision making are more appropriate than others. The three main frameworks discussed in the literature are:

- the information-processing model;
- the intuition model; and
- the cognitive continuum theory model.

We will explore these briefly as they relate to decision-making situations in which student nurses will be involved, and we will offer additional reading for more in-depth analysis of the use of each framework in nursing practice. We will explore these theories of decision making mainly in the context of clinical decision making rather than decision making generally, which is explored in **Chapter 2**.

Types of decision using the information-processing model

The information-processing theory of how we make decisions is based on how we manage information, obtained both in the short and long terms. You will start your nursing course with a store of information gathered from a number of sources and experiences. When you begin your course, you will be given new information, which initially you store in short-term memory; eventually, as you begin to learn additional information, this initial material will be stored as long-term memory (Aston et al. 2010).

An example that Aston et al. (2010: 7) offer is one from practice:

> '[W]hen a nurse assesses a patient for the first-time information is gained and immediately placed in short term memory. This then "triggers" certain cues that cause information retrieval from the long term memory.'

As you progress in your course of study, and as you acquire new knowledge and skills and, at the same time, gain experience in a variety of clinical placements, you will accumulate a great deal of information that will be retained in your long-term memory. Meeting a new situation for the first time, such as a new patient with a new life health history, may well 'trigger' this information that has, effectively, been kept 'in storage' until such time as it becomes apparent that it might be valuable in helping you to care for this new patient or in understanding his or her health problem—even though, on a personal level, he or she is new to you.

Of course, in nursing, as in any life experience, this one theory of how we use information is not the only way in which we can explain how we make decisions and, often, we use a number of different of theories to explain how we arrive at an action in nursing practice.

Types of decision using the intuition model

As with the information-processing theory of how we make decisions, our use of intuition in nursing is also based on information that is triggered from previous similar experiences. Benner et al. (1996: 142) talk about the 'expert practitioner', who makes decisions based on 'intuitive' links between what he or she is observing and what his or her subsequent response is.

Imagine, for example, that, as a student nurse, you observed during your first place-ment a situation in which a patient returning from theatre had collapsed and had to be resuscitated. His symptoms and physiological observations, which you had been in-volved in observing with your mentor, clearly indicated that he had suffered a heart attack following surgery, but he had no previous history of this possible outcome. In your third year, you are again on a surgical ward for a placement and are bringing a patient, who has had chest surgery, back from the operating theatre with a theatre nurse. You are observing the patient as you are returning with him from the recovery room and you note a change of face colour; he also begins to be agitated and complains of some chest pain. You take his pulse immediately and note that it is irregular. Your 'intuition' here tells you, based on your past experience in a surgical ward, as well as other experiences of the unexpected in other placements, that something is 'not right' with this patient. His clinical condition, as well as the fact that he is telling you about his chest pain, is confirming this 'intuitive' concern about this patient. A decision is required immediately: you are aware from that first experience of how quickly the patient could deteriorate. You decide (along with the qualified theatre nurse, who you have had to persuade, because she assumed from her knowledge of his chest surgery that his current problem resulted from that surgery) that he needs immediate care and agree to take him back immedi-ately to the recovery area of the operating department, where he can obtain immediate medical care and intensive monitoring of his observations. It is then diagnosed that he has, in fact, had a heart attack or myocardial infarction of some kind.

As you become more experienced after qualifying as a nurse, you will develop what could be called 'holistic knowing'—that is, the ability to see the 'bigger picture' (Benner et al. 1996), but making connections between what you see then and there, and your previous experience, to conclude that 'something is not right'. You might also say that you are using information stored in the memory, as well as previous experience and intuitive knowing, but these are very different types of decision making. Aston et al. (2010: 7) state that these two forms of decision making 'may be regarded as two ends of a spectrum as a means of decision making', but that, 'in reality, most nurses utilize a mixture of the two elements in their decision making'.

Types of decision using the cognitive continuum theory

Alongside the two other decision-making theories is what Thompson and Dowding (2002) call the 'cognitive continuum model of decision making', which represents a spectrum in which intuition decisions are at one end, while information processing and analysis is at the other (Aston et al. 2010). An example of a situation in which you have to use the latter type of decision making arises only when you are using evidence-based protocols, which Holland and Roxburgh (2012: 53) state are, 'in basic terms, steps laid down which are to be followed when making a decision for a range of situations'. They cite the examples of 'clinical procedure steps for infection control practice or a directive for a major disaster' and a study by Rycroft-Malone et al. (2009), which 'showed that qualified nurses used other kinds of information to help them make decisions even where protocol-based care was in place, and showed a range of decisions rather than following a standardized approach'.

Nursing practice is, it might be argued, an unpredictable environment, given that each patient and each nurse–patient encounter is unique and therefore unknown in terms of specific decision-making situations. However, even as a student nurse on his or her very first placement, you are able to draw on certain life experiences, on new information of various patient health problems, knowledge of physiology, and knowledge of how people live and of different cultural needs, as well as numerous other kinds of experiences and knowledge. An excellent example of how you can use this is in communicating with both patients and your peers who started their nursing course with you. Communicating with people is an essential requirement of being a nurse and the NMC requires all students to fulfil a range of communication competencies (NMC 2010).

....

⊕ Exercise

Consider how you would use intuition and information-processing models in communicating in the following situations.

1. A service user, who regularly comes to the school of nursing and whom you meet during a teaching session in the classroom, has come to talk to you about her experience of health care and has become very upset about her past experience in a certain local hospital whilst talking to you.
2. A student in your personal tutor group is very quiet during one of the teaching sessions about bereavement and dying. He is sitting next to you and you notice that he has begun to cry.

....

In the first situation, you may have considered intuitively that the woman must have had a 'bad' experience of health care to make her that upset and you may realize that you will need to make and communicate a decision regarding whether she needs to stop telling her story. You may also begin to recall that this local hospital she is talking about had been in the newspapers the previous year because of standards of care. Recalling this information will enable you to put the two issues together and to reassure the service user, as well as to ask another student to persuade the teacher to return to the classroom.

In the second situation, you may use intuition that 'something is not right' with this other student not only because he has started to cry during the teaching session, but also because you recall something that he said earlier to you about a parent's illness. Recalling this information, as well as the information that you have about the grieving process, will help you to make a decision to suggest quietly to the student that he might like to leave the class; you will also decide to offer to accompany him. (The teacher had already said, at the beginning of the session, that, not knowing the students' situations, she would understand if the session were to trigger some memories that may upset students and that she would fully understand if they were to have to leave the classroom—and that either she or a friend might accompany them.)

Decision making as a student nurse: the essential knowledge and skills

Given that nurses make decisions every day in practice about the care of their patients and clients, as well as decisions that affect their own personal and professional practice, it is important for you to consider how the student nurse learns to make decisions during his or her experience of learning to become a qualified nurse. The NMC (2010) makes it very clear that student nurses are expected to demonstrate their competence in decision making in relation to nursing practice, and that they are therefore expected to be taught and to learn these skills during their programme of study toward becoming a qualified nurse. This will involve learning in the clinical placement, as well as in clinical simulation teaching sessions, and will be underpinned by an evidence-based understanding of the decision-making theories. We all make decisions every day, from simplistic decisions regarding when to get up in the morning, to the more complex ones involving what do if you find a patient collapsed in his or her own home.

Box 1.1 draws together extracts from the NMC competencies in all fields of practice, 'Domain 3: Nursing practice and decision making'.

Box 1.1 Nursing and Midwifery Council competencies in all fields of practice

Domain 3: Nursing practice and decision making

Generic standard for competence

All nurses must practise autonomously, compassionately, skilfully and safely, and must maintain dignity and promote health and wellbeing. They must assess and meet the full range of essential physical and mental health needs of people of all ages who come into their care. Where necessary they must be able to provide safe and effective immediate care to all people prior to accessing or referring to specialist services irrespective of their field of practice. All nurses must also meet more complex and coexisting needs for people in their own nursing field of practice, in any setting including hospital, community and at home. All practice should be informed by the best available evidence and comply with local and national guidelines. Decision making must be shared with service users, carers and families and informed by critical analysis of a full range of possible interventions, including the use of up-to-date technology. All nurses must also understand how

(Continued)

Box 1.1 (Continued)

behaviour, culture, socioeconomic and other factors, in the care environment and its location, can affect health, illness, health outcomes and public health priorities and take this into account in planning and delivering care.

(NMC 2010: 17)

Field standard for competence (Adult)

Adult nurses must be able to carry out accurate assessment of people of all ages using appropriate diagnostic and decision-making skills. They must be able to provide effective care for service users and others in all settings. They must have in-depth understanding of and competence in medical and surgical nursing to respond to adults' full range of health and dependency needs. They must be able to deliver care to meet essential and complex physical and mental health needs.

(NMC 2010: 17)

Field standard for competence (Children)

Children's nurses must be able to care safely and effectively for children and young people in all settings, and recognize their responsibility for safeguarding them. They must be able to deliver care to meet essential and complex physical and mental health needs informed by deep understanding of biological, psychological and social factors throughout infancy, childhood and adolescence.

(NMC 2010: 44)

Field standard for competence (Learning disability)

Learning disabilities nurses must have an enhanced knowledge of the health and developmental needs of all people with learning disabilities, and the factors that might influence them. They must aim to improve and maintain their health and independence through skilled direct and indirect nursing care. They must also be able to provide direct care to meet the essential and complex physical and mental health needs of people with learning disabilities.

(NMC 2010: 35)

Field standard for competence (Mental health)

Mental health nurses must work with people of all ages using values-based mental health frameworks. They must use different methods of engaging people, and work in a way that promotes positive relationships focused on social inclusion, human rights and recovery, that is, a person's ability to live a self-directed life, with or without symptoms, that they believe is meaningful and satisfying.

(NMC 2010: 22)

Activity

Read the generic standard for all fields of practice and the specific one(s) for your field of practice reproduced in Box 1.1.

1. Consider, in particular, the knowledge and skills required to meet these parts of the 'Generic standard for competence' in Box 1.1:
    a. '*Decision-making* must be shared with service users, carers and families and informed by *critical analysis* of a full range of possible interventions, including the use of up-to-date technology.'
    b. 'All nurses must also meet more complex and coexisting needs for people in their own nursing field of practice, in any setting including hospital, community and at home. All practice should be informed by the *best available evidence* and comply with local and national guidelines.'
    c. 'They must assess and meet *the full range of essential physical and mental health needs* of people of all ages who come into their care.'
2. Use the field-specific standard competencies to determine one learning goal in relation to decision making in your next clinical placement. Ensure that you include the knowledge that you will need to learn with regards to the content of the competence statement.

In relation to the first point (a.), we can see that the action of decision making is to be shared with others and that the student is expected to critically analyse a range of possible interventions, including those involving technology. In essence, this competence involves evaluating the evidence base for decision making in relation to nursing interventions. *Critical analysis* of evidence is normally a requirement of an academic essay, which may focus on demonstrating that the student has reviewed the evidence on a topic or intervention, judged the positive and negatives involved, and supported his or her views with 'relevant literature and current research' (Duffy et al. 2009). Critical analysis is not about criticizing evidence; there must be an element of balance between the positives/benefits and the negatives/drawbacks, and you must use evidence to support your views. In the reality of clinical practice and making a decision such as whether one kind of nursing practice is more beneficial to the patient than another, nurses rely heavily on the fact that their decision will be based on an accurate and informed critical analysis and evaluation of the evidence that has been available to them.

In relation to the second (b.), we see here again the link between decision making and evidence-based practice (see **Chapter 3** for more detail). The NMC makes it clear that this has to be the *best* available evidence—ensuring again that this has been well evaluated by those providing it, whether it is a journal article, a book, or a policy document.

In the third point (c.), we can see the importance of assessing the needs of people, any decisions relating their care depending very much on the nurse's ability to assess their needs in the first instance and then to follow that with the ability to meet the person's 'essential physical and mental health needs'. This requires decision-making skills informed by knowledge of numerous health problems and underlying physical or mental causes, and, most importantly, how they are often interlinked in some way. We will see evidence of decision making in these areas in **Part 3** of the book, comprising those chapters that relate to specific decision making in the four fields of nursing practice highlighted in **Box 1.1**.

Once you have critically analysed the evidence available, you will then need to demonstrate how you decide on which information and evidence to use to inform your decision. This is where your critical thinking skills come into play—where you may have the best evidence available, but now have to decide on how best to use this to help the patient or client for whom you are caring. Applying best evidence cannot be undertaken in isolation from a range of other factors, such as care environment, your own skill set, any cultural factors that may impact on patient's needs, or the possible actions and decisions that may be required of other health care professionals. The nurse has to 'sift' through all of these factors in order to be able to base his or her decision on 'best' evidence. This sifting, or selecting, and making a judgement is critical thinking.

As a student nurse, you will more than likely question, when observing qualified nurses in practice, how and why they decide that a particular action is the best choice at one time, for example when undertaking oral hygiene of a patient, but then, in a similar situation the next day, make a completely different decision. In this situation, you are likely to find that the scenario and the evidence may remain the same—that is, how to undertake oral hygiene and what to use to clean the mouth—but that the patient is different (the first patient may have been elderly, while the second is young) and that multiple other factors are consequently different, leading to a different decision.

Critical analysis and critical thinking are therefore closely linked in terms of the skills that you need to acquire to become a competent practitioner. During your course of study in both university and practice placements, you will develop and integrate knowledge and experience, and you will achieve these skills by the end of your graduate programme. These two skills are also said to be indicative of a graduate education and Girot (2000), basing her views on a range of evidence, uses the terms 'problem-solve, reason logically, analyse information and form conclusions' as a way of defining critical thinking.

Clinical reasoning, clinical judgement, and decision making

We have notes that two other phrases used in conjunction with critical analysis and critical thinking are 'clinical reasoning' and 'clinical judgement'. Levett-Jones et al. (2010: 516) state that 'in the literature the term clinical reasoning, clinical judgement, problem-solving, decision making and critical thinking are often used interchangeably', but go on to cite Elstein and Bordage (1991), who view clinical reasoning as 'the way clinicians think about the problems they deal with in clinical practice. It involves clinical judgements (deciding what is wrong with the patient) and clinical decision making (deciding what to do)'.

We can begin to see a possible way of differentiating between all of these in terms of your learning to make decisions in clinical practice and, of course, in your other academic work. Clinical decision making can be seen as the end point at which you are seen to take an action of some kind based on the range of other skills deriving from critical thinking, critical analysis, clinical reasoning, and clinical judgement.

Levett-Jones et al. (2010: 516) offer a framework for clinical reasoning, called the 'five rights of clinical reasoning', based on the PhD study of Kerry Hoffman (2007), who explored how students and qualified nurses made decisions 'when caring for patients in an intensive care unit'. These initial thinking strategies that Hoffman had found were as follows:

- *describe the patient situation*
- *collect new patient information*
- *review information*
- *relate information*
- *recall knowledge*
- *interpret information*
- *make inferences*
- *discriminate between relevant and irrelevant information*
- *match and predict information*
- *synthesize information to diagnose or identify a problem*
- *establish goals*
- *choose a course of action*
- evaluate

(Levett-Jones et al. 2010: 561)

The 'five rights' of clinical reasoning in relation to the student nurse and how new or novice nurses can apply them are 'the ability to collect the right cues and take the right action for the right patient at the right time for the right reason' (Levett-Jones et al. 2010: 517). See Levett-Jones et al. (2010) for a diagrammatic view of the clinical reasoning process. See also their project website (<**http://www.newcastle.edu.au/project/ clinical-reasoning/resources.html**>) for further resources.

Tanner (2006) undertook a major review of the evidence on clinical judgement in nursing, on which she based 'an alternative model of clinical judgement'. She concluded that there were five key themes arising from this evidence:

1. *Clinical judgements are more influenced by what nurses bring to the situation than the objective data about the situation at hand*
2. *Sound clinical judgement rests to some degree on knowing the patient and his or her typical pattern of responses, as well as engagement with the patient and his or her concerns*
3. *Clinical judgements are influenced by the context in which the situation occurs and the culture of the nursing care unit*
4. *Nurses use a variety of reasoning patterns alone or in combination*
5. *Reflection on practice is often triggered by a breakdown in clinical judgement and is critical for the development of clinical knowledge and improvement of clinical reasoning*

(Tanner 2006: 204)

Conclusion

We can see, from an exploration of the evidence available to us with regards to definitions and explanations of what decision making entails as a qualified nurse, what a student nurse has to learn and what skills he or she has to gain to become an effective caring decision maker in practice. These skills have to be underpinned by an evidence base, not only in terms of the knowledge underpinning the rationales for decision making at any level, but also the increased importance of developing critical analysis and critical thinking skills in both theory and practice. These skills are essential, along with an in-depth knowledge of patient care situations and experiences, to developing clinical reasoning and clinical judgement skills, all of which underpin the effectiveness of decision making in nursing practice. Integrating what is learned in theory and clinical simulation environments with what is then experienced in the context of clinical practice will ensure the successful development of decision-making skills, allowing you to become the competent practitioner that you must be to become a registered graduate nurse.

We will be exploring many of these definitions and examples from practice in every part of the book. Further reading and resources will be identified to enable you to add to your knowledge according to your individual needs, as well as to help you to achieve your NMC competencies in all fields of practice.

References

Aston, L., Wakefield, J., and McGown, R. (eds) (2010) *The Student Nurse Guide To Decision Making In Practice*, Maidenhead: Open University Press.

Benner, P., Tanner, C., and Chesla, C. A. (1996) *Expertise in Nursing Practice: Caring, Clinical Judgement and Ethics*, New York: Springer.

Duffy, K., Hastie, E., McCallum, J., Ness, V., and Price, L. (2009) 'Academic writing: using literature to demonstrate critical analysis', *Nursing Standard*, 23(47): 35–40.

Elstein, A. and Bordage, J. (1991) 'Psychology of clinical reasoning', in J. Dowie and A. Elstein (eds) *Professional Judgement: A Reader in Clinical Decision Making*, Cambridge: Cambridge University Press, cited in Levett-Jones et al. (2010: 517).

Girot, E. A. (2000) 'Graduate nurses: critical thinkers or better decision makers?', *Journal of Advanced Nursing*, 31(2): 288–97.

Hoffman, K. (2007) 'A comparison of decision making by "expert" and "novice" nurses in the clinical setting: monitoring patient haemodynamic status post abdominal aortic aneurysm surgery', Unpublished PhD thesis, Sydney University of Technology, cited in Levett-Jones et al. (2010).

Holland, K. and Roxburgh, M. (2012) *Placement Learning in Surgical Nursing: A Guide for Students in Practice*, Edinburgh: Bailliere Tindall Elsevier.

Jones, R. A. P. (1996) 'Processes and models', in R. A. P. Jones and S. Beck (eds) *Decision Making in Nursing*, Albany, NY: Delmar, pp. 3–24.

Lasater, K. (2007) 'Clinical judgement development: using simulation to create an assessment rubric', *Journal of Nursing Education*, 46(11): 496–503.

Levett-Jones, T., Hoffman, K., Dempsey, J., Jeong, S. Y.-S., Noble, D., Norton, C. A., Roche, J., and Hickey, N. (2010) 'The "five rights" of clinical reasoning: an educational model to enhance nursing students' ability to identify and manage clinically "at risk" patients', *Nurse Education Today*, 30(6): 515–20.

Nursing and Midwifery Council (2010) *Standards for Pre-Registration Nursing Education*, London: NMC.

Rycroft-Malone, J., Fontenla, M., Seers, K., and Bick, D. (2009) 'Protocol-based care: the standardisation of decision making', *Journal of Clinical Nursing*, 18(10): 1490–1500, cited in Holland and Roxburgh (2012).

Standing, M. (ed.) (2010) *Clinical Judgement and Decision Making in Nursing and Inter-Professional Health Care*, Maidenhead: Open University Press.

Tanner, C. A. (2006) 'Thinking like a nurse: a research-based model of clinical judgement in nursing', *Journal of Nursing Education*, 45(6): 204–11.

Tappen, R. (1989) *Nursing Leadership and Management: Concepts and Practice*, 2nd edn, Philadelphia, PA: S. A. Davis Co., cited in Jones (1996: 3).

Thompson, C. and Dowding, D. (eds) (2002) *Clinical Decision Making and Judgement in Nursing*, Edinburgh: Churchill Livingstone.

Thompson, C. and Dowding, D. (eds) (2009) *Essential Decision Making and Clinical Judgement for Nurses*, Edinburgh: Churchill Livingstone/Elsevier.

Further Reading

Cameron, M. E., Schaffer, M., and Park, H. (2001) 'Nursing students' experience of ethical problems and use of ethical decision-making models', *Nursing Ethics*, 8(5): 432–47.

Gurbutt, R. (2006) *Nurses' Clinical Decision Making*, Oxford: Radcliffe.

Useful Links and Resources

<http://www.newcastle.edu.au/project/clinical-reasoning/resources.html>

The website of the Clinical Reasoning Project, University of Newcastle, Australia, includes a number of teacher resources, quizzes, and tests, as well as video material.

2

Making decisions as a student: decision-making opportunities

Deborah Roberts

The aims of this chapter are to:

➔ consider the principles of decision making in the context of undertaking a course of study;

➔ consider the various general decision-making situations that will impact on your learning to become a nurse;

➔ consider the type of decision that you will be required to make in relation to clinical placements and your role as a student nurse; and

➔ consider the different ways in which academic and practice staff can help you to achieve your goal of becoming a qualified nurse.

Introduction

This chapter introduces the underlying principles of decision making. You will be encouraged to consider decision making as a student in university together with decision making as a student nurse (see **Chapter 1**). In 2010, following a review of pre-registration nursing education, the professional body for nursing in the United Kingdom, the Nursing and Midwifery Council (NMC), published new *Standards for Pre-Registration Nursing Education*, including competencies that all students must achieve to qualify as a registered nurse. These competencies have to be met in four broad areas known as 'domains'.

1. Professional values
2. Communication and interpersonal skills
3. Nursing practice and decision making
4. Leadership, management, and team working

You will find reference to these domains throughout the book, and there will be an opportunity to learn how the competencies in each of these that relate to decision making can be linked to your clinical and university-based learning.

Decision making, problem solving, and clinical reasoning: what is the difference?

There are a number of terms that can be found in the literature that are often used interchangeably; you may see terms such as 'decision making', 'problem solving', 'clinical reasoning' or 'clinical judgement', and others used when writers are discussing how and why nurses respond to clinical situations in a particular way (see **Chapter 1** for more detail).

For example, Levett-Jones et al. (2010: 515) provide a helpful definition of clinical reasoning as 'the process by which nurses collect cues, process the information, come to an understanding of a patient problem or situation, plan and implement interventions, evaluate outcomes, and reflect on and learn from the process'. They also emphasize that a nurse's ability to develop these clinical reasoning skills depends on what they term as 'five rights'—that is, the nurse's ability 'to collect the right cues and to take the right action for the right patient at the right time and for the right reason'.

In the context of ensuring that any patient receives the best possible care, these 'five rights' are very appropriate, and indeed if one were to fail to pick up on the right cues and to take the appropriate actions in many clinical situations, the outcome may have serious repercussions for the nurse and the patient. We will be exploring some of the professional issues related to decision making in **Chapter 4**.

As we saw in **Chapter 1**, it is generally recognized that problem-solving skills and decision-making skills are not the same. Problem solving is a broader phase of the decision-making process, if it is used in decision making at all. The first stage might involve framing the issue as a problem—in other words, acknowledging that a problem exists. A problem must then be analysed (problem solving) before a range of actions to be taken is identified and a suitable solution selected from those identified (decision making).

Problem solving is a process through which you develop an understanding of the situation in order to make changes. Problem solving will involve intra-personal factors (your own motivations—to be a good person, for example), interpersonal factors (those that apply to others, such as a patient in pain), and extra-personal factors (perhaps in relation to your profession or institution), because all will have an impact on the outcome. People balance these factors in different ways and this is why people solve problems in different ways. Similarly, it is also why people make different decisions. Decision making is widely regarded to be a combination of interpersonal, technical, and cognitive skills. It is important to stress that decision-making skills do not develop by chance and that, as a student, you will have to develop your decision-making skills in readiness for taking decisions as a qualified nurse.

In order to start this process of developing decision-making skills generally, we can begin by looking at how we already use these in non-clinical situations.

Decision making as a student nurse

(1) Where am I now?

Life is full of decisions that must be made. However, for the most part, we do not really stop and think about these. In other words, these decisions could be said to be unconscious, or 'tacit'.

Try the following exercise.

....

 Exercise

Think about all of the decisions that you have made today. Write down the first ten of these.

After that, make a note against each as to what the outcome of the decision was and whether this was positive or negative. Decide why it was one or the other.

....

You might have come up with the following decisions:

● whether to press the snooze button on the alarm clock (perhaps more than once);
● whether to cancel the alarm altogether and go back to sleep;
● whether to get out of bed at all to begin your working day;
● whether to shower now or wait until later;
● whether to wash your hair in the shower;
● what clothes to wear;
● whether you need to wear formal shoes or trainers;
● what to have for breakfast;
● whether to take the bus or train, or drive to college; and
● whether to take an umbrella or only a waterproof jacket in your rucksack/bag.

Of course, you may not have considered any of these decisions at all and may have a completely different list, but when you begin to consider this type of decision making, it then becomes clear that we continually make decisions in our everyday lives without having to analyse them in any depth. We will, however, consider some of them more carefully than others, because they may have more serious outcomes than others. For example, deciding how much money to spend on a holiday or a new car could have an impact on your family budget or on your student grant funds for the rest of the academic year. Decision making is a highly complex activity and it is something that is particularly important in nursing practice.

Your decisions may also depend on your role at the time. We all adopt a number of different roles for different people all of the time; some are long-lasting and we adopt these roles for many years, such as 'daughter', 'brother', 'cousin', 'father'. Some roles are less permanent and we may occupy them for shorter periods of our lives, such as 'customer in a shop', 'patient at a "well woman" clinic'. Now that you have decided to become a nurse, you have assigned yourself another of these temporary roles: 'student nurse'. Just as in general life, there may be decisions associated specifically with becoming a student nurse.

⊕ Exercise

Think about how you will travel from where you live to university and to your placements. Make a note of both types of decision and consider what influenced those decisions.

You might have arrived at one or more of the following decisions:

- to walk to your (clinical) placement;
- to take the car to university;
- to take the bus to (clinical) placement if it rains;
- to take the car to university, but to try to find another student with whom to car share; and
- to take a taxi to (clinical) placement on bank holidays when there are few buses.

Your decisions about how you will get to university and placement will be personal to you. There will be a number of factors that you may have taken into account; you may have weighed up the 'pros and cons', and considered the financial implications of your decision. You may not, however, have used a framework or rules to guide your decision making.

(2) Decision making and becoming a student

The journey to being a student begins much earlier than your first day of university. In the first instance, what made you decide to become a nurse?

You have applied and been accepted onto a university pre-registration nursing programme, which will equip you with the knowledge, skills, and professional attitudes to be a qualified nurse in whichever field of practice you have elected to study. But how did you decide which university you would attend?

Perhaps you made some pragmatic decisions about attending whichever university was closest to where you live, or had placements that were close to where you live? On the other hand, you may have made a conscious decision to study away from your home town. You may have wanted to know whether individuals graduating from your university have found gainful employment. Perhaps you looked carefully at the facilities on offer at different universities and considered which would provide you with the best academic

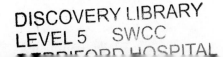

or pastoral support. You may have looked at what previous students have said about particular universities as part of the National Student Survey (**<http://www.thestudent-survey.com/institutions.html>**).

You will have weighed up a number of different factors that will have influenced your decision.

....

 Exercise

Think back to your reasons for choosing the university at which you are studying. Consider all of the information that you had to find, as well as any personal issues that you had to consider in making your decision. What major changes did you have to make in your life before starting the course, and how did these impact on others in your social and family groups?

....

Your course of study will take place in both the university and health care organizations such as the National Health Service (NHS).

(3) Being a student nurse at university

As a student nurse, you can expect to attend lectures at university on a regular basis. At the beginning of the programme, you might think that you will attend every lecture. However, there might be times when you decide not to attend. (You may even believe that you have a valid reason for not attending a particular session.) Do you think that there will be any consequences if you decide not to attend every lecture?

The NMC Standards (2010: 8) state that 'The programme can be no less than three years or 4,600 hours in length'. The NMC continues:

> Overall the programme requires 50 per cent theory (2300 hours) and 50 per cent practice (2300 hours), with some flexibility in each part of the programme ...
>
> There must be two progression points normally separating the programme into three equal parts. Progress in acquiring the competencies is mapped through the use of minimum progression criteria, based on safety and values (annexe 2), which the student must meet to progress from one part of the programme to the next. We set out minimum periods of practice learning towards the end of each progression point. The first progression point is normally at the end of year one. To pass the second progression point, normally at the end of year two, the student will need to demonstrate that they can be more independent and take more responsibility for their own learning and practice (annexe 2).

A nurse mentor who has completed specific preparation in assessing students is normally responsible for ongoing supervision and assessment in practice settings and in simulation. Other registered professionals who have been suitably prepared can supervise and contribute towards the assessment of nursing students. During a period of at least 12 weeks practice learning towards the end of the programme, a sign-off mentor (a nurse mentor who has met additional criteria), who is registered in the field of practice that the student intends to enter, makes a final judgement of competence (see Standards to support learning and assessment in practice (NMC 2008)). The evidence must show that the student is safe and effective in practice at the end of the programme.

(NMC 2010: 9)

What this means is that your university must demonstrate to the NMC that you have fulfilled this requirement in order for you to qualify as a nurse. In other words, you must have completed the requisite 4,600 hours of study, split equally between university and clinical practice, to complete your programme and qualify as a nurse. Therefore, whilst missing a lecture might seem fairly unimportant at the time, doing so could have an impact on your completion of these required hours.

Incidentally, the requirement of your university to account for the time that you spend on the programme also extends to the time that you spend on clinical placements. Therefore, if you are ever unwell and unable to attend either university or a clinical placement, it is important that you are aware of, and act in accordance with, your university's policy for reporting such absence. Similarly, you may be required to indicate your presence at lectures by signing a register, so that the university can maintain a record of your attendance.

Activity

What if you were to ask a friend to sign the register on your behalf, even though you will be absent from the session? What impact do you think this decision could have on your learning to become a qualified nurse?

Download the NMC Standards (2010) (see the link at the end of the chapter) and read through what will be required of you at these two key stages—in particular, the competencies that you are required to meet in relation to your professional behaviour and values. Discuss the implications with your personal tutor, who may already have this planned into your first meeting with him or her.

Table 2.1 Progression criteria relating to a decision not to attend a lecture

Areas associated with professional values and expected attitudes and behaviours towards people, their carers and their families		Related competency domains
13	Displays a professional image in their behaviour and appearance, showing respect for diversity and individual preferences.	Professional values Communication and interpersonal skills Nursing practice and decision making
...	...	...
17	Practises honestly and with integrity, applying the principles of The Code: Standards of conduct, performance and ethics for nurses and midwives (2008) and the Guidance on professional conduct for nursing and midwifery students (2009).	Professional values Communication and interpersonal skills Nursing practice and decision making

Source: NMC (2010: Annexe 2)

The NMC states that, by the first progression point, nursing students will demonstrate the progression criteria outlined in **Table 2.1**.

Not turning up to lectures could be construed as unprofessional behaviour, because doing so is part of the learning agreement that you will have signed as part of your learning to become a nurse. If you were to ask someone else to sign in on your behalf, both you and the person asked to do this would, in fact, be guilty of 'fraudulent behaviour'. (Developing professional values and acting like a professional nurse is fully discussed in **Chapter 5**.)

Being a student nurse at university will also involve attending other kinds of teaching and learning sessions in which you will be expected to engage in different kinds of group activity. This may involve undertaking group tasks and shared learning responsibilities. Some universities will use a particular teaching technique, called 'problem-based learning', which relies on all members of the group undertaking a range of tasks and roles so that they can learn about their course outcomes. You may be quite worried about working with other students, and at the same time wonder how and whether all students will put in the same amount of effort to complete the joint tasks in a timely fashion, to meet the learning outcomes of the work. You may even wonder whether you yourself will be able to contribute appropriately.

⊕ Exercise

You are part of a group of ten students who have been asked to prepare a presentation about your locality from a health perspective. You have all agreed which aspects of the presentation you are each responsible for and you are aware of what you are required to deliver. However, you have had a great deal of stress at home and you have been trying to work part-time at a local supermarket to ensure that enough money is available for your family's needs. The result is that you have not completed the work that you have agreed to do for the group presentation.

Consider the decisions that might be options here and make a note of what you think the consequences of your decisions might be.

You might have considered the following decisions:

- not to attend the session, but to phone in to say that you are unwell;
- to make a cursory attempt at something the night before the presentation, while aware that it will be of poor quality and quantity;
- to attend the session and to own up to the fact that you have not completed the agreed work; or
- because your friend, also completing the same exercise/work, is in another group with a different lecturer, to ask her if you can borrow her work to use in the session planned.

You might (quite rightly) be worried about letting your fellow students down by not completing the work. In addition, you should consider the impact of whether you are demonstrating the professionalism expected of a nurse. **Chapter 5** explores this in greater detail and will help you to understand what 'fitness to practise' means to you as a student nurse.

All four of these options have consequences and all four will have an impact on the rest of your group. The NMC is quite clear about students' responsibilities in terms of the levels of professionalism expected of them.

If you decide to ask your friend, you would be using someone else's work and claiming it to be your own. This is referred to as 'plagiarism' and includes:

- cheating in examinations, coursework, clinical assessment, or record books;
- forging a mentor or tutor's name or signature on clinical assessments or record books; or
- passing off other people's work as your own.

The NMC is very clear about the implications of plagiarism for your progression to becoming a qualified nurse. If you were to make this decision, you would bring your fitness to practise into doubt.

In addition, plagiarism is taken very seriously by universities and most have policies regarding such matters. So, before making any decision with regards to undertaking any kind of plagiarism, you should ensure that you are aware of what constitutes plagiarism and, more importantly, what the consequences might be for ignoring the rules. In some cases, you might receive a mark of zero for the assignment—or for the module as a whole. You may even be asked to withdraw from the course. Not being aware of the rules will not be a defence, so make sure that you fully understand your responsibilities as a learner.

(4) Being a student nurse in clinical practice

Your programme of nurse education in the UK is equally split between learning as a student in university, and learning as a student in (clinical) practice. Learning in practice means that you could be working in hospitals, nursing homes, general practitioner (GP) surgeries, patients' own homes, and other environments. Whilst in university, the typical learning day will be from 9 a.m. to perhaps 5 p.m. However, when learning in clinical practice, you will be expected to learn by working alongside other nurses—and this will mean undertaking to work different patterns of work periods, often known as 'off-duty' or 'working shifts'.

It can take a while to get used to working shifts in clinical practice, but it is important that, as a student nurse, you experience the 24-hour care of patients and clients. (It is, in fact, an NMC requirement that students undertake learning periods covering the whole 24-hour care period.) You will work alongside a qualified nurse, known as a 'mentor'. For more specific information concerning how to get the most out of your mentor, who takes responsibility for your overall learning experience in one given placement at a time, see Roberts (2010).

➕ Exercise

A family wedding, which has been planned for a long time, is scheduled to take place in the middle of your next clinical placement. The wedding is taking place at the other end of the country, and you would really like to have four days off over a long weekend so that you can travel and be at the wedding. Your family have made it clear that they expect you to attend, but you are unsure if you will be allowed the time off.

What factors might you take into consideration here that might inform your decision?

The following are three possible decisions that you might make:

- to say nothing to your mentor or the nurse in charge, but to phone in on the Friday morning pretending to be unwell;
- not to attend the wedding and to upset the bride and groom, not to mention your family members; or
- to talk to your mentor about your situation and ask for help.

Again, each of these options will have consequences. From the earlier examples in this chapter, you should now be fully aware of the consequences of pretending to be unwell and missing four days on placement, from an absence and a 'fitness to practise' perspective.

There may be other options open to you, such as putting in a request early enough to have those four days be your non-shift days for the one week and the next—that is a 'long weekend'. Generally, you will not be able to take the time off as annual leave or holiday, because these are normally set in a timetable for your three-year course of study. Talking to your mentor is the best option and he or she is likely to suggest requesting those days as non-learning days for the week.

The most important thing when making decisions of this kind is to plan ahead, and to discuss with the mentor your learning needs and any other issues such as booking 'days off' in advance. You will be required to meet the required hours per week of learning that your university expects of you, and that applies both in university and in the practice areas. These hours will be set for you and could be 35 hours a week of learning time (timetabled as lectures or seminars, or as self-directed study) in university and 37.5 hours a week in practice. The way in which those hours are expressed will be through the timetable in university and, of course, through what is often known as the 'off-duty rota' in practice.

Decisions about yourself and how you learn

Being a student nurse will undoubtedly mean lots of new learning—but have you ever stopped to consider how you learn, or what your experiences of learning have been? Your view may depend on whether you are a mature student who has done other things, including work, before undertaking a pre-registration nursing programme. Indeed, you may have wanted to be a nurse for a long time, but delayed starting this programme until your children are at an age at which you feel you can commit to the programme, or you may have waited until your children left home. You may, in fact, feel as though you have never stopped learning—that is, you might be accessing the pre-registration nursing programme after completing further education. Whatever the case, it is important that you really think about the way(s) in which you learn. This will help you to make decisions about getting the most from your experiences throughout the pre-registration programme.

Activity

Access the following websites and undertake the tests provided; this will give you a range of ideas about how you learn best.

<http://www.vark-learn.com>

VARK is a 'guide to learning styles'. It explores how we process information.

<http://www.campaign-for-learning.org.uk/aboutyourlearning/whatlearning.htm>

The Campaign for Learning website provides a questionnaire to help you to determine your learning style.

<http://www.infed.org/biblio/b-learn.htm>

This website will give you supporting information about learning styles and draws on Honey and Mumford's (2000) learning style theory to help you to work out what kind of learner you are.

<http://www.engr.ncsu.edu/learningstyles/ilsweb.htm>

This 'Index of Learning Styles Questionnaire' helps you to determine your learning style.

(Continued)

Once you know what your learning style is or preferences for learning are, start to make some decisions about how you might use this information to make the most out of all of the learning opportunities that there will be in both university and clinical practice. You might want to write these as action plans, which specify how you use the knowledge you have about how you learn. Decision making, as you can see, becomes an integral part of your learning to become a nurse.

It might be useful, for example, for you to know whether you have a preference for *visual* or *kinaesthetic* processing. If your style is visual, you might prefer to watch a demonstration of a nursing intervention several times before undertaking it yourself under supervision. If you prefer to process information in a kinaesthetic form, you might prefer being 'hands-on', or 'doing', right from the start and experimenting yourself with the nursing intervention. There might be opportunities for you to experiment in this way in the safety of a skills lab before you meet real patients.

If, however, you have assessed yourself as being a *reflector*, you might prefer to sit back in lectures and think about things carefully, rather than to contribute your ideas to the discussion without thinking. If you are an *activist* (very much like having a kinaesthetic processing preference), you might prefer to learn by doing and being physically involved.

 ## Top Tips

Start a learning diary

A learning diary allows you to reflect regularly on significant experiences associated particularly with your (university) learning. It will help you to become more aware, and to acknowledge what you have learned and how you have progressed. Stopping to think about how you learn will help you to identify issues or problems associated with your learning, and, by so doing, you will be able to consider ways in which you can overcome these. This, of course, may already be a requirement for some of you, and will form part of your personal and professional development activities (see Burton and Ormrod 2011; Hart 2010).

Use a soft-backed, small exercise book (not loose paper) to record your thoughts. Get started by spending no more than five minutes every day (rather than half an hour once a week). Review what you have written once a week (perhaps on Sunday evening, when you might also be planning your coming week's activity). Also, review what you have written more generally every month or two, to gain an overview and to discover patterns of learning or issues that are similar in your decision-making practice.

Write about activities at both university and clinical placement, such as situations or experiences involving decision making that went well or were difficult, and try to think about why this was the case. Consider any unexpected problems or issues, such as a particular drug calculation maths problem or your technique on giving an injection. Think about habits that you have noticed in yourself or others (which have some relevance) in relation to learning: for example, do you take a long time before jotting down notes about the assignment that you have to write? Remember to use the learning diary to think about how you feel about the way in which you are doing things, looking at understanding, clarity of thought, strength of actions, and awareness. How effective are you, for example, in using feedback from others and achieving goals (such as assignment deadlines, finding information in a library, or even keeping a learning diary)?

Write down anything else that feels important to you—even though you may not understand its significance at the time. This will help you to learn from your successes, as well as your mistakes, making it more likely that you will use what you have learned next time, rather than to 'make the same mistakes', or to 'fall back on old habits' or practices.

Keeping a learning diary gives you an opportunity to plan concisely what you want to do and what you want to change, and to make some plans as to how you will go about addressing these issues.

As part of your nurse education programme, you will often be expected to write about your experiences of caring for patients. In particular, you will have to demonstrate that you have understood the theories and principles that you have been taught in class, and that you are able to apply these to your practice as a student nurse. It is important that you write about your experiences and patient encounters in such a way that places and people cannot be identified.

⊕ Exercise

Try to write a few lines about your last visit to your doctor (GP) or the dentist, the reasons for your visit, and what took place. Some of you may also have been hospital patients at some time before starting your course.

How would you feel if someone else were able to read this account?

You may have found it quite difficult to write about this experience without naming the GP, the practice, the hospital, or without providing personal information.

Standard 7 (NMC 2010) reads as follows: 'People can trust the newly registered graduate nurse to protect and keep as confidential all information relating to them.'

By the first progression point at the end of the first year, you must be able to demonstrate the following three skills and behaviours:

> 1 *Applies the principles of confidentiality.*
> 2 *Protects and treats information as confidential except where sharing information is required for the purposes of safeguarding and public protection.*
> 3 *Applies the principles of data protection.*
>
> (NMC 2010: 111)

You will need to write about clinical examples in such a way that you ensure that anonymity is maintained. For example, you could write:

> I was recently allocated to a general surgery ward at a large general hospital in the north-west of England. It was here that I nursed a patient who I shall call 'Mr Jones' in order to maintain and ensure patient confidentiality in accordance with the NMC Code.

It will be becoming apparent, then, that there will be many decisions for you to make in order to succeed in becoming a qualified nurse. In the next section, we will consider the principles of decision making in nursing practice.

Decision making in nursing practice

This section of the chapter will explore decision making in relation to nursing practice, beginning with an exploration of the types of decision making that are commonly experienced by nursing in all fields of practice. The decisions that you were asked to consider in the first exercise in this chapter might be termed 'everyday', or 'lifestyle', decisions, but how might decision making for nursing be different?

 Exercise

Imagine the first hour on your next placement. Write down the first three decisions that you might have to consider.

You may have noted the following decisions:

- what you might discuss with your mentor when you meet him or her for the first time;
- whether to ask any questions about the patients/clients for whom you will be caring that day;
- whether to ask for your 'shift hours' as soon as the morning report has been given about the patients for whom you will be caring that day.

Now think about your answers to this exercise in relation to the following types of decision described in **Chapter 1**. What do you have to consider before making the decision to act on any of these three decisions? Your answers will very much depend on whether you have considered the 'cues' either in the context of care or what is actually happening around you, what evidence that you are 'picking up' about whether it is a good time to be asking any of the questions, how busy your mentor is, what is happening with the patients in your care, whether your shift hours might simply be read from the 'off-duty' rota on the notice board in the staff area of the ward or community office.

The frequency of decision making in nursing practice is dependent on five interrelated factors:

- the clinical environment;
- the patients that can be found within that environment;
- the nurse's perceptions of his or her clinical role;
- operational autonomy; and
- the degree to which he or she sees himself or herself as an active and influential decision maker (Thompson et al. 2004).

The study by Thompson et al. (2004) demonstrates three levels of what they term 'decisional complexity', meaning that nurses often have to respond to clinical situations with quick decisions and often have to make decisions that are complex. Their study showed that student nurses take more time to collect information on which to base their decisions, whereas experts spend less time seeking information to reduce uncertainty in decision making. So, remember that decision making as a student nurse may not be as fluid and speedy as the decision making that will emerge as you develop your expertise; the time that you take to collect information on which to base your decisions is important and should not be underestimated.

Conclusion

This chapter has explored the general principles of decision making and it has related these to decision making as a student nurse. The chapter has provided an introductory overview of the types of decision that you might have to make as a student nurse in university and in clinical practice. It is not possible to cover every eventuality, but the following chapters will offer you other options. The main consideration is that, when you are unsure of making a decision that could possibly have serious consequence, you should always ask someone first—whether that is a personal tutor or programme leader in the university, or your mentor and other practitioners in your placements.

Your ability to make the right decisions will develop over the course of your learning journey to becoming a qualified nurse. It is important that you make these decisions based on best evidence available at the time and, of course, that your decisions do no harm to yourself, to your colleagues, and most importantly to those patients and clients for whom you will be learning to care and with whom you will be working.

References

Benner, P., Tanner, C., and Chesla, C. A. (1996) *Expertise in Nursing Practice: Caring, Clinical Judgement and Ethics*, New York: Springer.

Burton, R. and Ormrod, G. (2011) *Nursing: Transition to Professional Practice*, Oxford: Oxford University Press.

Giuliano, K. (2003) 'Expanding the use of empiricism in nursing: can we bridge the gap between knowledge and clinical practice?', *Nursing Philosophy*, 4(1): 44–52.

Hart, S. (ed.) (2010) *Nursing Study and Placement Skills*, Oxford: Oxford University Press.

Honey, P. and Mumford, A. (2000) *The Learning Styles Questionnaire*, Maidenhead: Peter Honey Publications.

Levett-Jones, T., Hoffman, K., Dempsey, J., Jeong, S. Y., Noble, D., Norton, C. A., Roche, J., and Hickey, N. (2010) 'The "five rights" of clinical reasoning: an educational model to enhance nursing students' ability to identify and manage clinically "at risk" patients', *Nurse Education Today*, 30(6): 515–20.

Nursing and Midwifery Council (2008) *Standards to Support Learning and Assessment in Practice*, London: NMC.

Nursing and Midwifery Council (2010) *Standards for Pre-Registration Nursing Education*, London: NMC.

Roberts, D. (2010) 'How you will learn in practice', in S. Hart (ed.) *Nursing Study and Placement Skills*, Oxford: Oxford University Press, pp. 137–56.

Thompson, C., Cullum, N., McCaughan, D., Sheldon, T., and Raynor, P. (2004) 'Nurses, information use, and clinical decision making: the real world potential for evidence-based decisions in nursing', *Evidence-Based Nursing*, 7(3): 68–72.

Further Reading

Aston, L., Wakefield, J., and McGowan, R. (2010) *The Student Nurse Guide to Decision Making in Practice*, Maidenhead: Open University Press.

Banning, M. (2007) 'A review of clinical decision making: models and current research', *Journal of Clinical Nursing*, 17(2): 187–95.

Gurbutt, R. (2006) *Nurses' Clinical Decision Making*, Oxford: Radcliffe.

Useful Links and Resources

<http://standards.nmc-uk.org/PublishedDocuments/Standards%20for%20
pre-registration%20nursing%20education%2016082010.pdf>

The NMC (2010) *Standards for Pre-Registration Nursing Education*.

<http://www.newcastle.edu.au/project/clinical-reasoning/resources.html>

The website of the Clinical Reasoning Project, University of Newcastle, Australia, includes a number of teacher resources, quizzes, and tests, as well as video material.

3

Using evidence for decision making

Thérèse Leufer and Joanne Cleary-Holdforth

The aims of this chapter are to:

➔ explore the importance of using evidence to underpin nursing decisions;

➔ explore how student nurses can use evidence to underpin their decision making in practice; and

➔ ensure that student nurses can identify how evidence can be used to meet nursing competencies involving decision making.

Introduction

By now, you have read lots of information on the principles of decision making and why this is so important for you in your nursing practice. It will be invaluable to you as you progress in your nursing career to know how to make decisions in and about nursing practice, including knowing:

- when to make these decisions;
- when decisive action is required;
- when to call a doctor;
- when to withhold a particular medication; and
- when to recommend an alternative nursing intervention.

It is equally imperative that you understand why you are making the decisions that you are making and where you might go to find the information that you need to underpin these decisions.

The Nursing and Midwifery Council (NMC), in its *Standards for Pre-Registration Nurse Education* (2010), specifies clearly the competencies that are required upon completion of a nursing programme for entry to the NMC professional register. In its competency framework, four key areas ('domains') are identified, one of which is 'Nursing practice and decision making', demonstrating unequivocally the emphasis and importance that the NMC places on the role of the qualified nurse in decision making. This domain statement is presented in **Box 3.1**. Specific requirements relating to this domain can be found in **Parts 2** and **3** of this book.

Box 3.1 Domain 3: Nursing practice and decision making

1 All nurses must use up-to-date knowledge and evidence to assess, plan, deliver and evaluate care, communicate findings, influence change and promote health and best practice. They must make person-centred, evidence-based judgements and decisions, in partnership with others involved in the care process, to ensure high quality care. They must be able to recognize when the complexity of clinical decisions requires specialist knowledge and expertise, and consult or refer accordingly.

(NMC 2010: 26)

In addition, the NMC stipulates, in relation to specific knowledge and skills, that 'all nurses must apply knowledge and skills based on the best available evidence indicative of safe nursing practice' (NMC 2010).

It also offers guidance to programme providers on the 'Essential Skills Clusters' (NMC 2010)—that is, additional sets of skills ('clusters' of skills set around specific areas of nursing practice) required to be attained by student nurses at specific points during their programme. The Essential Skills Cluster that is relevant to the use of evidence to underpin practice decisions is the 'Organisational aspects of care'. Within this cluster, there are a number of descriptors listed that are related to this area, as listed in **Table 3.1**.

This chapter will discuss how the use of evidence-based practice can help you to best support your clinical decisions and help you to avoid making the incorrect or inappropriate decision. We will provide you with a practical framework and approach to clinical decision making that will enable you to find appropriate, relevant evidence on which you can rely to help you to make the decision in the first instance, and also to qualify your rationale to defend that decision as it impacts on the delivery of patient care. Developing skills to find best evidence, to then use it when deciding on the best possible outcome for the patient, will be highlighted throughout the chapter.

Table 3.1 Essential skills cluster: organizational aspects of care

Second progression point	Entry to the register
	9(14) Applies research based evidence to practice
10(4) Actively seeks to extend knowledge and skills using a variety of methods in order to enhance care delivery	
	14(9) Act as an effective role model in decision making, taking action and supporting others
	16(3) Bases decisions on evidence and uses experience to guide decision making

Source: NMC (2010)

Evidence-based practice: what is it?

So what is evidence-based practice (EBP), and why are we reading and hearing about it more and more? Evidence-based practice has gained global momentum amongst various health care professional groups since its original inception in the early 1970s and indeed has been described as 'a movement' by Rees (2010). Jolley (2010) considers EBP to be a process, perhaps indicating its dynamic and evolving nature. Evidence-based practice is a holistic approach to care delivery that places the individual patient at its core. It is far more than simply the use of research; it is a partnership between inter-professional clinicians, patients, and the best available evidence to optimize patient outcomes (Cleary-Holdforth and Leufer 2009). While this may seem like a convoluted definition to describe what EBP is, it is, to put it more simply, an approach to patient care that takes into account key influential factors to help us to make a decision regarding the patient's care. These factors include:

- patient preference or opinion;
- the nurse's/clinician's experience and expertise; and
- relevant evidence from research, expert reports, or significant organizations.

All of these factors contribute to a patient care decision that will provide the best results for the patient.

In the not-too-distant past, it could be argued that nursing care was considered to be based on ritual and/or medical consultant/ward sister personal preferences. The individual nurse's expertise and/or experience were not always influential in the decision making around patient care. In our view, there were practices that were not always grounded in 'sound evidence' and decisions about clinical care were often not queried in terms of why practice was changed, or indeed why it was not.

The routine rubbing of alcohol into patients' buttocks in the belief that such rigorous friction, coupled with a drying substance, would somehow prevent the development of pressure sores; the topical application of egg white and oxygen therapy to established pressure sores, in the belief that this would heal them; the use of 'Edinburgh University Solution of Lime' (Eusol) for wound de-sloughing, which has courted immense controversy over the years (Tingle 1990): these are a just a few practices that the authors and some of your tutors would have witnessed in their respective student nursing training.

Activity

1. Visit a relevant database (examples can be found later in the chapter) and undertake a search for current evidence in relation to the following practices:
   (a) the routine rubbing of alcohol into patients' buttocks to prevent the development of pressure sores; and
   (b) the use of Eusol for wound de-sloughing.   *(Continued)*

2. Reflect on the nature of the evidence that may have been used to underpin these practices in the past. Consider alternatives at the time in the 1960s and 1970s.
3. Read Clark, M (2002) 'Pressure-reducing cushions: the Cinderella of support surfaces?', *Nursing Times*, 98(8): 59, available online at <http://www.nursing-times.net/pressure-redistributing-cushions-the-cinderella-of-support-surfaces/200372.article>.
4. Consider the evidence provided and why the author concluded that there was insufficient evidence on which to base best practice decisions in the use of pressure-relieving cushions in pressure ulcer prevention.

Questioning such practices was not encouraged, and the culture and historical background of nursing largely compelled nurses to 'follow orders'. Evidence-based practice, on the other hand, actively encourages questioning, and values ongoing accessing and critical appraisal of evidence in the scrutiny of practice and the pursuit of improved patient outcomes. Jolley (2010) suggests that EBP enables the 'weeding out' of ineffective practices, and the identification and implementation of improved practice. This highlights the importance of ensuring balance in your thinking when considering the rationale underpinning patient care. While the evidence supporting a particular practice may not be highly visible, or indeed readily accessed, this does not always mean that this particular practice is not based on evidence or indeed does not have value in patient care. Indeed, Rees (2010) comments that EBP is concerned with the standard of care delivery and how evidence is used to inform clinical decisions. It is a process comprising seven easy-to-follow steps that guides the nurse from his or her initial question about an aspect of patient care through to the most appropriate decision for the individual patient, and its implementation, evaluation, and dissemination (see **Table 3.2**).

Table 3.2   Steps of the evidence-based practice process

0	Cultivate a spirit of enquiry
1	Ask the burning clinical question in PICOT format
2	Search for and collect the most relevant best evidence
3	Critically appraise the evidence
4	Integrate the best evidence with your own clinical expertise, and patient preferences and values, in making a practice decision or change
5	Evaluate outcomes of the practice decision or change based on evidence
6	Disseminate the outcomes of the evidence-based practice decision or change

Source: Melnyk and Fineout-Overholt (2011: 10)

Activity

For an example of a practice that appears to be without a sound evidence base (traditional Chinese healing), but which nonetheless demonstrated positive benefits for patients with cancer, read Xu, W., Towers, A.D., Li, P., and Collett, J. (2006) 'Traditional Chinese medicine in cancer care: perspectives and experiences of patients and professionals in China', *European Journal of Cancer Care*, 15(4): 397–403.

We will now explain some of the key terms associated with EBP.

Evidence

The meaning of the word 'evidence' in its broader application is 'something which provides ground for belief or disbelief' (*Collins Concise Dictionary and Thesaurus* 1995: 318). However, the evidence to which we refer is that which should be used to underpin practice in the nursing context. So, in this context, what is 'evidence'? Melnyk and Fineout-Overholt (2011: 4), long-time active proponents of EBP, define evidence as 'a collection of facts that are believed to be true'. They further classify evidence into 'internal' and 'external' evidence, which describe evidence generated from practice and that generated from research, respectively. Examples of evidence from practice (internal evidence) and how it can be generated include outcomes from quality improvement projects involving patients, clinical audits on various aspects of patient care delivery, and the results of outcomes measurements on patient interventions (Black and Jenkinson 2009; McDonnell et al. 2007; Melnyk et al. 2006; Thompson 2003). External evidence, on the other hand, is generated by conducting formal research studies or clinical trials to investigate or explain a particular phenomenon relating to an aspect of patient care, for example a research study to explore the experience of 'phantom pain' in patients who have undergone a below-knee amputation (Desmond et al. 2008), or a study to test the relationship or link between cigarette smoking and lung cancer (Center for Disease Control and Prevention 2011). These are just two examples of how evidence that can be used to answer clinical questions contributing to decisions about patient care is generated from research. From this, it is clear that there is more than one source of evidence on which we can draw to underpin practice. In fact, Rycroft-Malone (2004) suggests that there are four sources of evidence: research; clinical practice/experience; patients; and the context of the evidence.

   With the spotlight placing emphasis on different types of evidence used to underpin decision making, the role of the patient in shared decision making is brought into clear focus (Pearson et al. 2007). Patients, as the recipients of the care being decided upon and delivered, must, wherever possible, be central to the decision-making process regarding their care. Individual patient preferences/idiosyncrasies will influence care planning and decisions. It is imperative that the individual patient's voice is heard and influences the care that he or she receives if the true meaning of 'individualized patient care' is to be realized.

Individualized care is a two-way process, and it is imperative that the patient is involved in decisions affecting his or her health and well-being (Rycroft-Malone and Bucknall 2010). It is not only about the nurse perceiving the patient as an individual human being; while this is important, it is also about the nurse hearing and respecting the very valuable and pertinent perspective and input offered by the patient. Patients (and their carers) are a very significant, but perhaps underutilized, resource—but a resource input that EBP recognizes and values as a core component in its approach to underpinning decision making in patient care delivery.

The final source of evidence described by Rycroft-Malone is the context in which one is practising. Decision making about patient care cannot happen in a vacuum or in isolation from the real-life situation that is the context of care. Crucial factors, such as the particular setting, patient profile, ward philosophy and culture, and the organization of care delivery in the particular facility, among others, can potentially have a huge influence on how decisions are reached about patient care delivery.

The process of evidence-based practice

As previously indicated, the process of EBP comprises seven clear steps (Melnyk and Fineout-Overholt 2011: 10), which were outlined in **Table 3.2**.

On close consideration of the steps of the EBP process, you may, like us, feel that there appear to be similarities between these and the steps of the nursing process (Holland and Rees 2010)—that is, assessment, planning, implementation, and evaluation. Indeed, this is clearly reflected by the NMC (2010) in its *Standards for Pre-Registration Nursing Education*, 'Domain 3: Nursing practice and decision making', in which the NMC refers to what could be described as a 'trinity' of essential elements—namely, the nursing process, clinical judgement and decision making, and evidence-based practice—and the importance of all three being interwoven in nursing practice in order to 'influence change and promote health and best practice' (NMC 2010: 17). This is not too distant from the overall priorities identified by Lord Darzi in his review of the National Health Service (NHS), which emphasizes the need to 'create an NHS that helps people to stay healthy' (Department of Health 2008: 2). As nurses working at the forefront of health care systems, it is crucial that this too must be the primary goal of your practice.

As you may appreciate from the nursing process, before you embark on delivering any patient care, you must first take a step back, assess the patient and the situation, and ask yourself: 'What does my patient need? What is the best course of action in this context?' This, in essence, is the first step on the road to clinical judgement and decision making. Many theories exist in relation to clinical judgement and decision making, as you discovered in **Chapter 1**. However, in order for practice to be influenced by such theories, thereby, arguably, narrowing the theory–practice gap, such theories need to be 'accessible, understandable, relevant and applicable' (Standing 2011). In other words, they need to make sense to the nurse in the context of his or her practice. With this in mind, we will offer Standing's explanations of both clinical judgement and clinical decision making, to ensure that we have a shared understanding of what these terms mean.

Clinical judgement and decision making

Clinical judgement, as defined by Standing (2011: 7), is 'informed opinion (using intuition, reflection and critical thinking) that relates observation and assessment of patients to identifying and evaluating alternative nursing options'. It can be argued that intuition, reflection, and critical thinking are largely subjective and invisible in nature. Intuition, in particular, has attracted much debate and controversy over the years with regard to its legitimacy as a basis for decision making, and indeed a general consensus on what exactly it is (Benner and Tanner 1987; Cioffi 1997; Pellegrino 1979; Thompson and Dowding 2009). However, it is clear from Standing's definition that decision making is underpinned by a combination of these subjective components with the more tangible, explicit, or 'scientific' components, such as patient physiological observations and assessment. Standing goes on to emphasize how clinical judgement is applied in the clinical decision-making process 'to select the best possible evidence-based option to control risks and address patients' needs in high quality care for which you are accountable' (Standing 2011: 8). This process of clinical judgement and decision making clearly draws on a number of key components, such as intuition, reflection, and critical thinking, to underpin your decision regarding the best course of action to implement for the patient(s). The steps of EBP, as outlined in **Table 3.2**, facilitate these processes by helping you to ask the relevant patient care question, and guiding you to and through the available evidence, thereby enabling you to select the best available evidence to underpin your patient care decisions with confidence.

As is clear from **Table 3.2**, there is a logical order to the steps of the EBP process. This process, similar to the nursing process, will always begin with a question: to get the information required on which to base your clinical judgement and decision, you need to ask the right question. The information that you are seeking should ideally be the best-quality evidence that is available to ensure that you are delivering the best possible care. To this end, there are levels of evidence that are ranked in order of their quality and potential usefulness to the practitioner. These levels are well documented and are frequently referred to as a 'hierarchy of evidence'.

Once you have gathered the best-quality, most relevant evidence that you can access, and that you feel will help to inform your clinical judgement and decision making, you must determine its usefulness by assessing its quality. Thereafter, depending on the conclusions that you reach about the quality of the evidence that you have collected, which involves critical review (Holland and Rees 2010), you will be in a position to decide what to do next. There are two possible outcomes at this point.

First, you may find that the evidence that you have reviewed indicates that the standard of care that you are currently delivering is, in fact, consistent with best practice, in which case you will simply continue with this practice. Alternatively, this evidence might point towards the need to change or amend existing practice in some way, to ensure that it is the most up-to-date care and is consistent with international standards, for example. When a change in practice is implemented, it is imperative that the results are closely monitored and measured to ascertain whether the desired results were in fact achieved. This is akin to the 'evaluation' step in the nursing process, and provides the opportunity to take stock—to determine whether your decision making and subsequent actions have yielded the desired outcome(s) for your patient or practice. If the desired outcomes have not been achieved, then it is essential that you return to the first step of the EBP process, reflect carefully on the desired outcome(s), and revisit the components that underpinned your clinical judgement (perhaps your intuition or critical thinking around aspects of the situation) in coming to that decision(s). It may at this point be necessary to rearticulate your clinical question either with a different focus or level of specificity; indeed, a new question may even be warranted. In this way, this EBP process, similar again to the nursing process, can in fact become cyclical in nature and application.

Activity

Read Stewart, E. (2006) 'Nursing guidelines: development of catheter care guidelines for Guy's and St Thomas", *British Journal of Nursing*, 15(8): 420–5, which considers one example of how the process of EBP is operationalized or implemented in practice—in this instance, to underpin the development of new catheter care guidelines.

The steps of evidence-based practice for decision making

Decision making plays an integral role in nursing practice and, during the course of your career, you will find yourself in situations in which you need to make different types of decision, which might be classed as 'routine', 'responsive', and 'emergency'. It has been suggested that different types of decision are informed by different types of judgement (Standing 2011; Thompson and Dowding 2009).

- In the *routine* situation, you can take a more considered approach to decision making, because you have the luxury of time and access to resources including senior colleagues, policies, protocols, and, if necessary, published materials that you can consult to help you to reach decisions and to plan or deliver care.
- There will equally be situations that will arise that you did not anticipate or foresee and for which therefore have not planned—that is, the *responsive* situation. This type of situation requires more of a 'thinking on your feet' approach and draws on a variety of judgement types, involving personal experience, peers, the patient(s), and the local context.
- The third type of situation that you may encounter in practice is an *emergency* decision, which demands prompt and confident decision making in an effort to maximize the outcome for the patient, as far as possible. This situation can take you very much by surprise, because not only is it unplanned, but it is also usually spontaneous and urgent in nature, requiring immediate action. In this type of situation, decisions are often underpinned by intuition and reflection in action (Schon 1983), and the benefit of peers as a resource, together with the patient and the local context, or any combination of these. (Reflection will be discussed in more detail in **Chapter 4**.) This type of decision needs to be made very quickly and almost 'without thinking'. Thompson and Dowding (2009) describe such decisions as 'fast and frugal'.

The examples outlined in **Table 3.3** illustrate some of the many situations in which you may find yourself throughout your nursing career that will require you to make a decision. With some of these situations, you will not have much time to make decisions; in others, such as the routine example, you will be in a position to make a less

Table 3.3 Examples of types of decision in practice

Routine decision making	As a student nurse, you are concerned that the taking and recording of patient physiological observations that are scheduled for 10 a.m. are often not undertaken at this specified time, as a result of other activities on the ward, including meeting patient hygiene needs, doctors' rounds, medication rounds, patients leaving the ward for investigations/procedures, and so on. You consider the possibility of suggesting a trial change to this policy, bringing the 'observations round' forward to 8 a.m. from 10 a.m. You have seen this on another ward, and it seemed to allow for more timely and efficient monitoring and recording of observations. This reflective, perhaps intuitive, clinical judgement may need to be further supported by consulting other sources, including peers, patients, and indeed the relevant literature on this subject, in order to underpin any decision making on this issue.
Responsive decision making	As a qualified nurse, you are undertaking a drug round during which you are required to administer prescribed medications to your patient. Your patient, who normally accepts his medications without hesitation, refuses to take his medications on this occasion. You will need to respond to this situation by thinking on your feet and deciding the best course of action to address this unanticipated scenario.
Emergency decision making	Such situations could include a patient collapsing, the outbreak of a fire requiring evacuation, cardiac arrest, or a confused aggressive patient, to mention only a few. You will need to respond immediately and appropriately to such situations.

spontaneous, more considered decision. Evidence-based practice plays a vital role in all types of clinical decision making. Therefore it is imperative to develop the skills required to engage in the process of EBP, to foster good judgement and decision-making practices as you progress in your nursing career.

We will now explore each of the seven steps of the EBP process, reaffirming the importance and relevance of evidence in making decisions and the types of evidence most suitable.

> ### Reflective activity
>
> Before reading the seven steps involved in EBP, consider the types of decision outlined in Table 3.3. In relation to each decision type, reflect on your experiences in clinical practice and provide examples of each decision type that you have encountered. Consider also how these decisions were made and what 'evidence' informed or facilitated them.

Step 0 Cultivate a spirit of enquiry

While this step may seem more like an organizational, rather than an individual, strategy, it is important to acknowledge that we all have our part to play in this regard. A culture and environment in which practitioners are happy and comfortable with raising questions about the current standard of care or current practice is evidence that a spirit of enquiry exists in an organization. When management and senior staff are seen to welcome questions about current practice and suggestions as to how patient care could perhaps be enhanced, there is an 'openness' to enquiry and to embracing of EBP. It is important also that management is seen to support practitioners in the development of skills necessary to advance this spirit of enquiry, and indeed to operationalize EBP through practice development initiatives. From the individual practitioner's perspective, it is prudent that he or she embraces this culture, and avails himself or herself of every opportunity offered to develop necessary knowledge and skills to enable him or her to contribute actively to the spirit of enquiry and to enhancing patient care.

As a student nurse, you will be working and learning alongside your mentors and other practitioners, who should be actively encouraging this spirit of enquiry.

> ### Reflective activity
>
> Based on your knowledge and understanding of EBP and what you believe a spirit of enquiry to be, reflect on your clinical placements to date and ask yourself whether you have seen or experienced a spirit of enquiry in any of these environments.
>
> *(Continued)*

1. What do you believe characterizes a spirit of enquiry in a clinical setting?
2. How is a spirit of enquiry demonstrated in your current placement?
3. Discuss with your mentor how you can gain an opportunity to develop your EBP skills in practice in order to meet the NMC competencies that will be part of your final placement assessment. (This will be determined as well by your own university practice assessment requirements and whether you are being assessed at the main progression points.)

Step 1 Asking the important clinical question

As we noted earlier in the chapter, the starting point in this process is the articulation of an important clinical question. Where do these questions emerge from? Many of them arise from day-to-day practice, when nurses find themselves asking questions such as:

- 'Is there not a better way of doing this?'
- 'There must be a better dressing for this wound that will speed up healing and reduce the frequency of dressing changes?'
- 'I wonder if music therapy might reduce my patient's anxiety levels or episodes of challenging behaviour?'

All of these require the nurse to make a decision of some kind. The nurse is prompted to ask these kinds of questions because he or she is engaging actively in patient care every day and is motivated to do his or her best for his or her patients. Other questions will be triggered by specific conditions, particular patient needs, or experiences encountered, or indeed when new or alternative interventions are being considered.

To develop these ideas or questions that emerge from practice to a point at which they can be articulated, or 'asked aloud', so that the process of answering them might begin, it is important that you begin by writing something down (whether on paper or electronically), giving due consideration to the specifics of what you are asking and the question to which you need an answer. This is the start of the very essential step in EBP in which you need to develop a very clear question relating to the aspect of practice about which you wish to enquire. This important clinical question needs to be one that will readily allow you to search for information or evidence on databases, for example, and also one to which you can realistically find an answer. In other words, this question needs to be 'searchable' and 'answerable', so that it will yield, or allow you to get to, the information that you need. There are established frameworks in existence that will help you to construct questions in this way, including the PICOT question framework (see '**Asking your question using the PICOT format**').

Activity

Consider a question about an aspect of your practice that you have considered, which relates to patient care. Such questions are the starting blocks for clinical judgement and decision making in practice, and are crucial if clinical practice is to evolve and improve over time. Indeed, your question may also be one that you are asking toward completing an assignment, or even a dissertation or systematic literature review.

1. In your own words, construct and write down the question* that you wish to ask.
2. Enter the keywords or key terms from your question into a database of your choosing (for example, the Cumulative Index to Nursing and Allied Health Literature, or CINAHL) and see how many 'hits', or results, you obtain from your search.
3. Determine how many of these 'hits' appear irrelevant or unrelated to the question that you asked.

*You will need to refer to this question again after we look at the PICOT format for framing clinical questions (see 'Asking your question using the PICOT format').

The clinical question needs to be well considered, focused, and reasonably specific. If you have taken sufficient time to make notes or to prepare in the manner indicated, you will be well on your way to framing your question.

To newcomers to the EBP process, this step can at first seem arduous and time-consuming. However, the time spent developing a well-articulated clinical question is time well spent and pays significant dividends in the end. If this step is rushed, or not given the necessary time and attention, it is likely to lead to an unrefined search, resulting in an abundance of literature accrued, presenting an unmanageable task, leading to an unsuccessful outcome. This becomes disheartening and frustrating, and the practitioner runs the risk of abandoning the search for an answer to his or her clinical question as a result.

As a student, it is important that you understand how clinical questions are asked, so that when you are evaluating evidence to underpin practice (engaging in critical review), you can at least have an understanding of how the question asked by the researchers was determined and ultimately how the findings of their investigations answered it.

To help you with the process of writing a searchable answerable question, there are many evidence-based question framing tools that exist (Craig and Smyth 2007; Dawes et al. 2005; Gerrish and Lacey 2006; Melnyk and Fineout-Overholt 2005). These will help you to break down your question, to identify the important elements of your question, and guide you in terms of where to place due emphasis in your question. Melnyk and

Fineout-Overholt (2011) recommend using a tool known as the 'PICOT format' to enable you to ask your clinical question by considering the specific components of interest.

Asking your question using the PICOT format

The 'PICOT format' comprises five individual components or elements, all of which need to be clearly articulated within a question. Each element must be clearly identified to enable the drafting or construction of a searchable, answerable question. Each of the five letters of the mnemonic denotes a component of the question that should be considered when writing it.

The components, as described by Melnyk and Fineout-Overholt (2011: 30), are:

- **P**—*population*, or disease, of interest (details such as age, gender, ethnicity or co-morbidity, and intellectual disability or mental health considerations);
- **I**—*intervention*, or range of interventions, or issue of interest (such as therapy, exposure to disease, risk behaviour such as smoking, or an issue of interest to the clinician);
- **C**—*comparison* intervention or issue of interest (alternative therapy, placebo or current practice, absence of disease or absence of risk behaviour, such as non-smoking);
- **O**—*outcome* of interest (expected outcome from therapy, for example improved/ faster healing or reduced episodes of challenging behaviour, or improved self-belief/self-esteem levels); and
- **T**—*time* involved to demonstrate an outcome (for example, the time expected for a smoking cessation intervention to work—that is, for the smoker to stop smoking).

Within the PICOT framework, several question templates are provided to help you to construct your specific clinical question. These include templates for intervention-type questions, prognosis-type questions, diagnosis-type questions, and meaning-type questions, and include templates such as that supplied by Melnyk and Fineout-Overholt (2011). It must be stressed at this point that no one question template is appropriate in every context. For example, if the clinical question were to relate to a relatively unexplored area of nursing practice such as the experience of women living with multiple sclerosis, there would be no 'intervention' as such, nor would you be comparing it with anything; the focus would be purely on the 'issue' that is the lived experience of this one group of women. In this instance, the meaning template would be more appropriate and useful, because the 'I' component relates to an issue of interest rather than an intervention and the 'C' component (comparison) is not important or relevant.

PICOT offers a clear framework for developing a clinical/practice question, which in turn facilitates the best way in which to search and find the evidence, through ensuring that the right 'keywords' are formulated and then used in the database searches.

To demonstrate how a framework such as PICOT can help you to articulate your clinical question in a useable way (which will be searchable and answerable), we will use an example of a clinical question that might be raised.

Constructed or written before applying the PICOT format, the question might be phrased as follows:

> How often should patients who are confined to bed rest be moved from their previous position?

If we look at this question more closely, it will become apparent that it lacks the detail and specifics needed to guide and execute a strategic and fruitful search. In its current state, if you were to go to the computer to search relevant databases, you would be highly likely to yield thousands of 'hits' or results on the general area of 'patients confined to bed'. The majority of this information would be irrelevant, would lack quality, and would not provide an answer to your question. Remember: the computer is only as useful or helpful as the 'instructions' that you give it.

The importance of taking the time necessary at this stage to get your question right cannot be overemphasized. In the example question that we have provided, the crucial elements that can immediately be seen to be absent are the **I**ntervention, **C**omparison, **O**utcome, and **T**ime.

The only element that is visible to some degree is the **P**opulation. However, even this lacks focus and specific details to help to guide a meaningful search. The information that is provided here in relation to the population is 'patients who are confined to bed', which is very vague. There is no indication of age profile, setting, or presenting and/or underlying diseases to help to refine the question and the subsequent search.

Here is an example of how this question may be asked in a more focused and refined manner:

> For patients who have had a stroke and are confined to bed (*P*), what is the effect of two-hourly turns (*I*) on skin integrity (*O*) compared with four-hourly turns (*C*) over the course of one month (*T*)?

As you can see, the question now contains all of the elements of the PICOT format, which are needed in this particular scenario to produce a clearly defined question in preparation for step 2 of the EBP process.

In the case of some clinical questions or in particular settings, it may not always be essential or warranted to include the **C**omparison element. For example:

> How do mothers (*P*) who have been diagnosed with post-natal depression (*I*) perceive the impact of this condition on their ability to bond with their babies (*O*) in the first year post delivery (*T*)?

Similarly, it may not always be appropriate to include a Time dimension, as the following sample question illustrates:

> Are service users of mental health services (*P*) who have a history of (deliberate) self-harm (*I*) at increased risk of completed suicide (*O*) compared with individuals without a history of (deliberate) self-harm (*C*)?

Irrespective of the clinical question that you are asking or the clinical background from which you are coming, it is important to invest the time and effort into formulating a good question that has a clear structure and contains the necessary elements of the PICOT format. As previously indicated, the Comparison and Time elements of this format do not always need to be included. However, the Population, Intervention, and Outcome elements must always be included and clearly defined. Formulating your questions strategically using a framework like PICOT renders the next step of the EBP process infinitely easier, as we will now see.

Activity

Consider the question that you previously asked (in your own words) about an aspect of your field-specific practice.

1. Using the PICOT format outlined above, rethink your question and the key terms that you might now use.
2. Enter these (perhaps revised) key terms into a database of your choosing (for example, CINAHL) and see how many 'hits' or results you obtain from your search on this occasion.
3. Ascertain, at a glance, how many of these 'hits' appear irrelevant or unrelated to the question that you asked on this occasion.
4. Have you found any difference in the quantity and/or quality of the results that you have obtained second time around (that is, by using the PICOT format)?

This exercise will also help to develop your evidence-searching skills, which are essential to most types of academic assignment, which are underpinned by an evidence base, as we will now see.

Step 2 Search for and collect the most relevant best evidence

The type of evidence that you need will be determined by the clinical decision that needs to be made, for example whether it is how to manage the anxiety of patients undergoing

Table 3.4 Factors to consider when undertaking a search for evidence

What is the nature of the decision to be made?	Is it a clinical problem/an issue with a real patient focus? Is it an assignment requirement, e.g. a hypothetical scenario?
Is there a time constraint/urgency involved in this decision?	
What kind of evidence do I need?	For example, do I need to consult research or evidence-based practice guidelines or local policy? Do I need quantitative or qualitative evidence? What contribution can peers offer to this decision? What patient-related factors need to be considered?

general anaesthetic pre-operatively or how to manage the pain control needs of patients post-operatively. There are a number of questions that you may wish to ask yourself in advance of conducting your search. These are essential questions that you should ask to point you in the right direction to obtain the evidence necessary to underpin the necessary clinical decision. A sample of such questions is presented in **Table 3.4**.

Good planning and developing of that initial evidence-searching question is essential for *effective* decision making when searching the relevant databases or other possible web-based resources. It is important to have a well-articulated, searchable, answerable question prior to consulting these databases—but some of you reading this chapter may already have been asking the question: what can be classed as a 'database'?

Example of databases commonly used include:

- the Cumulative Index of Nursing and Allied Health Literature (CINAHL);
- the Excerpta Medica Database (Embase);
- The American Psychological Association's PsycINFO;
- Medline;
- Scopus;
- the Database of Abstracts of Reviews of Effects (DARE);
- the Cochrane Library; and
- Dissertation Abstracts Online (DAO).

It may be worth noting at this point that an invaluable resource in this area is the subject librarian in your library, who can help to guide you through the activity of searching relevant databases in the most efficient way possible.

Activity

In your clinical placement, find out whether there is a library in the area. This could be a library in the training and education centre in a hospital or community health centre, or the main town library.

Make a point of visiting the library early on in your placement (discuss doing so with your mentor first), and find out what resources are available and what access to resources is available to you as a student nurse.

In addition to these databases, there are several excellent web-based resources to guide you through the process of undertaking the search for the most relevant and best available evidence. In order to do this, you will need to input keywords or key terms to the database to commence your search. The benefit of having structured your clinical question using a format such as PICOT is that you immediately have to hand the words within your question that can serve as these key search terms to steer your database search.

Similar to Step 1, planning and conducting your database search may initially seem challenging or perhaps even unexciting. However, it too offers significant outcomes, particularly when you become more proficient and you start to find that your searches yield highly relevant, good-quality evidence with the 'hits' (that is, the number of articles/pieces of evidence that result from the search) numbering in the single digits rather than the hundreds or thousands that can result from poorly steered searches.

Holland and Rees (2010) recommend a number of useful resources (references, further reading, and useful websites) from the Online Resource Centre that accompanies Holland and Rees (2010) (see the end of the chapter for the link to this site) as tools to assist you in your search for, and retrieval of, evidence to underpin your decision making. A selection of these can be found in **Table 3.5**.

Now that you have collected your evidence, the next step is to decide on its quality and usefulness to your context in answering your question. In other words, will the information that you now have to hand provide answers that will help you in your decision making regarding the care of your patient? To answer this question may, at this stage, seem quite a daunting task. Perhaps a good place to start is to understand what is meant by the terms 'evidence' and 'quality evidence' in the context of this searching and reviewing activity.

A common perception is that if evidence is to be deemed to be of 'good quality', it must be derived from robust scientific research in hospitals or laboratories, such as clinical trials involving experimental approaches—perhaps a *clinical trial on a new drug to ascertain its effects and/or side effects*. However, quality evidence exists in many different guises

Table 3.5 Useful resources

<http://ebn.bmj.com/cgi/content/extract/3/3/71>	Cullum (2000)
<http://missinglink.ucsf.edu/lm/EBM_litsearch/case1page.html>	University of California Regents School of Medicine (2010) 'Searching the literature for evidence-based medicine'
<http://www.nottingham.ac.uk/nursing/sonet/rlos/studyskills/lit_search_advanced/>	University of Nottingham School of Nursing and Academic Division of Midwifery (2008) 'RLO: Advanced literature searching—Choosing databases' This site was developed as part of a funded initiative to set up a number of Centres for Excellence in Teaching and Learning (CETLs) throughout England. This one focuses on 'Reusable objects'.
<http://www.tripdatabase.com/>	Trip database

Source: Holland and Rees (2010: 65–6)

and includes studies, for example, that are not experimental in nature, such as an exploration of the *experience of parenting a child who has a profound intellectual disability*.

You will notice a clear difference in the focus, and indeed the type, of results that you might expect to emerge from these two respective examples. This is largely as a result of the different approaches used to answer different types of question and can be loosely grouped into two particular research approaches: quantitative and qualitative research.

The nature of the question being asked will often dictate the most appropriate research approach to obtaining the information (data) needed to answer the question and ultimately to make a decision in practice.

In the case of the drug trial, for example, clear decisive, unbiased data/results collected from large numbers of subjects are needed to answer the questions being asked. This data must be objective and must not be influenced by individual/group opinion, interests, or experiences. This quantitative approach may appear somewhat impersonal as a result of its precision.

However, this is equally where its strengths lie in answering those questions that are best tackled using this approach. There are minimal margins for error in this type of research, because drugs can potentially cause significant harm to patients, or at the very least may have little or no therapeutic effect.

On the other hand, the data required to answer the question concerning the experience of parenting a child with a profound intellectual disability is a very different kind of data.

This qualitative data, for example, focuses on the life experiences of particular individuals from their personal perspectives. Therefore this data must be personal in nature and is usually collected in person directly from smaller numbers of participants, who have direct experience of the phenomenon of interest (in this case, parents of children with a profound intellectual disability). It is the personal viewpoint of the participants that yields the answer to the question posed in the first instance. This personal account is what gives this approach to research its strength and uniqueness.

Activity

With respect to each of the questions listed below, answer the following.

1. What is the nature of the question being asked?
2. Do I need quantitative (such as numerical data) or qualitative (more narrative-type data) evidence?
3. Do I need to consult expert authorities, research, EBP guidelines, or local policy?
4. What contribution can professional peers offer to this decision?
5. What patient-related factors need to be considered?
   (a) Does education about contraception reduce unwanted pregnancies in young people who live in socially deprived areas?

(Continued)

(b)   Why do young people who live in socially deprived areas have a higher incidence of unwanted pregnancies?

(c)   What are the perceptions of young people living in socially deprived areas of
unprotected sex and contraceptive use?

Whether the evidence that you have collected is qualitative or quantitative in nature, you will still need to ascertain its quality and usefulness. To help you with this, there are tools known as 'hierarchies of evidence' (see **Clinical judgement and decision making**'), which present different types of evidence in ranked order of their quality and which a number of EBP proponents recommend (Cleary-Holdforth and Leufer 2008; Gerrish and Lacey 2006; Guyatt and Rennie 2002; Melnyk and Fineout-Overholt 2011). Many of the hierarchies available combine quantitative and qualitative evidence together in a single hierarchy. Holland and Rees (2010) advocate the use of a hierarchy that combines both qualitative and quantitative evidence to help when making a judgement about the quality and usefulness of the evidence that you have collected. An example of such a hierarchy is that developed by the Joanna Briggs Institute (see **Figure 3.1**), which is based in Australia.

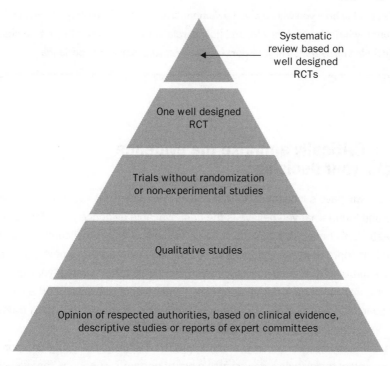

Systematic
review based on
well designed
RCTs

One well designed
RCT

Trials without randomization
or non-experimental studies

Qualitative studies

Opinion of respected authorities, based on clinical evidence,
descriptive studies or reports of expert committees

Figure 3.1 Example of a hierarchy of evidence. *Note:* RCT = randomized controlled trial. Reproduced from Holland K and Rees C (2010) *Nursing: Evidence-Based Practice Skills*, with permission from Oxford University Press.

Using this hierarchy, you can then map your respective pieces of evidence against the appropriate hierarchy and determine at what level of evidence each piece can be rated. This will be undertaken in advance of critically appraising your evidence to determine each piece's usefulness and potential contribution to answering your question, and there may, in fact, be some pieces of evidence that you can discard at this point before ever taking the time to critically appraise them. (See Holland and Rees 2010: ch. 7 for critical review frameworks for quantitative and qualitative research studies.)

Activity

The NMC (2010: 44) Generic Standard for Nursing Practice and Decision Making includes a competence which states that 'All practice must be based on current evidence and up-to-date technology'.

1. Review the hierarchy presented in *Figure 3.1* and consider how this can help you to achieve the above competence.
2. During your next placement, identify an area of practice that you will use to help you to demonstrate how you meet this competence when being assessed by your mentor.
3. Determine how you will be able to demonstrate that you have gathered this evidence, what the evidence is, and how it relates to the area of practice chosen. (Include the evidence in your portfolio of practice learning experience.)

Step 3 Critically appraise the evidence to make your decision

By now, you will have successfully formulated a relevant clinical question to your area of practice and found what you believe is the best available evidence with which to answer this question. You may also be in a position to discard any evidence of lesser quality or which is inappropriate for the focus of your clinical question. The next step—that is, critically appraising the evidence that does have merit for answering your question— may at first appear to be a daunting prospect. However, if you have used a clear strategy for searching and finding, and then choosing, the best evidence, then it does not have to be as challenging as it may first appear.

There are many ways in which you can approach this task, but using an appropriate critical appraisal tool will provide you with a list of pertinent questions that you need to answer in respect of your evidence. (An example of one of these for either a qualitative or quantitative study can be found in Holland and Rees 2010.)

> ## Activity
>
> Access these tools and review the different sections to be considered for critical review of the evidence that you have found and which you consider appropriate for answering the question that you have written. (It is not the purpose of this chapter to focus on this in detail, because we are considering how the evidence base itself is important for decision making.) Consider in particular how the review questions help you to determine:
>
> - whether the results of the study are valid (*validity*);
> - what the results are (*reliability*); and
> - whether the results will help you in caring for your patients (*applicability*).

It is evident from the considerations listed in this activity that a reasonable level of research knowledge, including the principles and process of both qualitative and quantitative research approaches, is needed in order to understand what is being asked in each and to be able to answer them. It will therefore be prudent to consult a good research textbook and to have one with you when engaging in critical appraisal.

Cleary-Holdforth and Leufer (2008: 45) state that 'Answering these questions enables nurses to ascertain the value of a given study in their day-to-day practice, thereby enabling them *to make informed decisions* about patient care in the clinical setting'.

> ## Activity
>
> - Consider an aspect of nursing care from the field of nursing practice in which you are particularly interested, for example oral hygiene.
> - Search for two articles on your chosen area, one qualitative and one quantitative. Using the critical appraisal tools that are accessible at the Online Resource Centre accompanying Holland K and Rees C (2010) (see the end of the chapter for the web link), try to undertake your own preliminary critical appraisal of these articles.
> - When you have completed this exercise, reflect on how the critical appraisal tools helped you in making sense of your chosen articles.
> - What was your final decision on the value of these papers for helping you to understand some of the evidence available on the chosen topic?
>
>   * Note that this is a good exercise to undertake for those of you who will be completing an assignment involving a similar exercise or a possible dissertation in your final year of study.

Step 4 Integrate the best evidence with your own clinical expertise, and patient preferences and values, in making a practice decision or change

At this stage, having critically appraised your evidence, you will now be in a position to decide on one of two options: either the evidence will indicate that the current practice in your clinical setting is consistent with other national or international standards, in which case you will continue with this practice and no change in practice will be warranted; or the evidence may indicate that your practice is not entirely in keeping with national or international standards, in which case some change in practice may be needed. (It is important to highlight here that, as a student nurse, you will not yet have ultimate decision-making authority and will need to liaise closely with your assigned mentor and relevant peers.)

So what do you do if the evidence appears to indicate that a change in practice is warranted? Consider the following scenario and possible learning experience that you could encounter in clinical placement.

⋯⋯

 Exercise

A recently completed audit in the care setting in which you are working has demonstrated a stark increase in reported medication errors in the previous calendar year. This is a cause for serious concern amongst the multidisciplinary team (MDT) members working within the area. A working group comprising members of this team has been set up to discuss the findings and to consider how best to tackle this problem. You are invited to attend, because your mentor is a member of the working group.

Reflecting on the definition of EBP and its core elements, consider the types of evidence that may be helpful in addressing this problem and informing the eventual decision making and outcome for patient care.

⋯⋯

Evidence-based practice is a holistic approach to care delivery that places the individual patient at its core. It is far more than research utilization alone and is a partnership between inter-professional clinicians, patients, and the best available evidence to optimize patient outcomes (Cleary-Holdforth and Leufer 2009).

When an appropriate course of action has been agreed and decided upon, it is imperative that a collaborative approach is employed and that key steps, such as education initiatives to inform practitioners as necessary, are taken in order to ensure a smooth transition in the adoption of the change in practice. Consideration must also be given at this stage to how the outcomes of the implemented change will be measured and with what these outcomes will be compared, to ascertain if patient care has benefited or if standards have improved as a result.

Reflective activity

Consider your role as a student nurse who has just undertaken and completed an assignment for which you searched, obtained, and critically appraised evidence on an aspect of nursing practice.

On a subsequent clinical placement, you find that qualified nurses in that area are engaging in practice that is contrary to what you found (through your assignment) to be the best available evidence. On reflection, how might you, as a student, address this difference in practice?

Discuss possible options with your mentor.

Step 5 Evaluate the outcomes of the practice decision or change based on evidence

Having implemented the change in practice that was deemed necessary based on the evidence obtained and reviewed, it is essential subsequently to measure the outcomes or results of this change. Outcomes measurement can take many forms and consider many aspects. Some examples of outcomes measurement can include patient satisfaction surveys, decreased cost of care or length of stay, physiological measures (for example, blood pressure, aerobic fitness, reduced infection rates, or improved wound healing rates), psychological measures (for example, levels of anxiety, quality of life, levels of depression), functional improvement (for example, improved gait or ambulation, return to independence), or nursing retention, improved staff morale, or job satisfaction.

The purpose of doing this is threefold. In the first instance, you want to determine whether the outcomes of the decision to change practice in your workplace mirror the outcomes of the same change documented in the evidence. Second, evaluating the outcome will allow you to inform future decision making around nursing practice and patient care in the aspect of care in question. If the outcomes are positive or if the desired outcomes have been achieved, then clearly the decision will be taken to continue with this new practice for as long as it continues to work or until new evidence recommends a change from this practice. Alternatively, if the outcomes are not as expected and the desired results of the change in practice have not materialized, it will be essential to investigate why this is the case. This may then involve further re-examination of the initial questions and further evidence being required to ensure successful decision-making outcomes.

Top Tips

It is worth noting that, in advance of undertaking an assignment or dissertation that requires you to ask or answer a clinical question, it is important to consider what the nature of the question is and the outcome or end result for which you are looking. This will help you to articulate your question, and to plan and direct your assignment.

Step 6 Disseminate the outcomes of the evidence-based practice decision or change

In order to maximize the learning that has been achieved through the EBP process that has led to and informed the implementation of a change in practice, it is imperative that this learning experience and its outcome is shared with as many interested parties as possible. To this end, nurses, including student nurses, can and should make efforts to disseminate the results of their endeavours so that other practitioners can learn from them and, in turn, many more patients can benefit from this work. Examples of how and/or where nurses can disseminate their work include 'in-house' study days, journal clubs, conference presentations (both poster and oral presentations), and professional publications. Although a daunting prospect, many students are now engaging in these, either on their own, or with their mentors or tutors.

Activity

Read Holland, K. and Rees, C. (2010: 248–85) on how students can disseminate their learning, including how to present the findings of their work.

Consider how you would present your work to the other students in your seminar group. See the Online Resource Centre that accompanies Holland and Rees (2010) for examples (see the web link at the end of the chapter).

Conclusion

This chapter has focused on the value and importance of evidence-based practice (EBP) in any decision making involving patient and client care. It has examined all aspects of what is required to determine that this evidence is the best available, including developing your searching and critical review skills, as well as how these can help you to achieve the necessary NMC (2010) Standards and competencies relevant to your stage of your learning, and eventually those essential for becoming a registered nurse. Making clinical judgements and decisions that enhance and support effective patient care outcomes, as well as the way in which that care is holistically delivered, will depend on the underpinning knowledge and practice evidence that you, as this future qualified nurse, will use.

References

Benner, P. and Tanner, C. (1987) 'How expert nurses use intuition', *American Journal of Nursing*, 87(1): 23–31.

Black, N. and Jenkinson, C. (2009) 'Measuring patients' experiences and outcomes', *British Medical Journal*, 330: 2495.

Center for Disease Control and Prevention (2011) 'State-specific trends in lung cancer incidence and smoking: United States, 1999–2008', *Morbidity and Mortality Weekly Report*, 16(60): 1243–7.

Cioffi, J. (1997) 'Heuristics, servants to intuition, in clinical decision making', *Journal of Advanced Nursing*, 26(1): 203–8.

Clark, M. (2002) 'Pressure-reducing cushions: the Cinderella of support surfaces?', *Nursing Times*, 98(8): 59.

Cleary-Holdforth, J. and Leufer, T. (2008) 'Essential elements in developing evidence-based practice', *Nursing Standard*, 23(2): 42–6.

Cleary-Holdforth, J. and Leufer, T. (2009) 'Evidence-based practice: sowing the seeds for success', *Nurse Education in Practice* (Guest Editorial), 9(5): 285–7.

Collins Concise Dictionary and Thesaurus (1995) Glasgow: HarperCollins.

Craig, J. V. and Smyth, R. L. (eds) (2007) *The Evidence-Based Practice Manual for Nurses*, 2nd edn, Edinburgh: Churchill Livingstone Elsevier.

Cullum, N. (2000) 'Users' guide to the nursing literature: an introduction', *Evidence-Based Nursing*, 3(3): 71–2.

Dawes, M., Davies, P., Gray, A., Mant, J., Seers, K., and Snowball, R. (2005) *Evidence-Based Practice: A Primer for Health Care Professionals*, 2nd edn, Edinburgh: Elsevier Churchill Livingstone.

Department of Health (2008) *High Quality Care for All: NHS Next Step Review Final Report* (the Darzi Report), London: HMSO.

Desmond, D., Gallagher, P., Henderson Slater, D., and Chatfield, R. (2008) 'Pain and psychosocial adjustment to lower limb amputation amongst prosthesis users', *Prosthetics and Orthotics International*, 32(2): 244–52.

Gerrish, K. and Lacey, A. (eds) (2006) *The Research Process in Nursing*, 5th edn, Oxford: Blackwell Publishing.

Guyatt, G. and Rennie, D. (2002) *Users' Guides to the Medical Literature*, Chicago, IL: American Medical Association Press.

Holland, K. (2010) 'Dissemination of evidence: writing for publication and presentation of learning activity', in K. Holland and C. Rees (eds) *Nursing: Evidence-Based Practice Skills*, Oxford: Oxford University Press, pp. 246–85.

Holland, K. and Rees, C. (2010) *Nursing: Evidence-Based Practice Skills*, Oxford: Oxford University Press.

Jolley, J. (2010) *Introducing Research and Evidence-Based Practice for Nurses*, Harlow: Pearson.

McDonnell, N., Kwei, P., and Paech, M. (2007) 'A disposable device for patient-controlled intravenous analgesia: evaluation by patients, nursing and medical staff', *Acute Pain*, 9(2): 71–5.

Melnyk, B. M. and Fineout-Overholt, E. (eds) (2005) *Evidence-Based Practice in Nursing and Healthcare: A Guide to Best Practice*, Philadelphia, PA: Wolters Kluwer Health/Lippincott, Williams & Wilkins.

Melnyk, B. M. and Fineout-Overholt, E. (2006) 'Consumer preferences and values as an integral key to evidence-based practice', *Nursing Administration Quarterly*, 30(1): 123–7.

Melnyk, B. M. and Fineout-Overholt, E. (eds) (2011) *Evidence-Based Practice in Nursing and Healthcare: A Guide to Best Practice*, 2nd edn, Philadelphia, PA: Wolters Kluwer Health/ Lippincott, Williams & Wilkins.

Melnyk, B. M., Feinstein, M. F., Alpert-Gillis, L., Fairbanks, E., Crean, H. F., Sinkin, R., Tu, X., Small, L., Gross, S., and Stone, P. (2006) 'Reducing premature infants' length of stay and improving parents' mental health outcomes with the COPE NICU program: a randomised clinical trial', *Pediatrics*, 118(5): 1414–27.

Nursing and Midwifery Council (2010) *Standards for Pre-Registration Nursing Education*, London: NMC.

Pearson, A., Field, J., and Jordan, Z. (2007) *Evidence-based Clinical Practice in Nursing and Healthcare: Assimilating Research, Experience and Expertise*, Oxford: Blackwell Publishing.

Pellegrino, E. D. (1979) 'The anatomy of clinical judgements', in H. T. Engelhardt, Jr, S. F. Spicker, and B. Towers (eds) *Clinical Judgement: A Critical Appraisal*, Dordrecht: D. Reidel, pp. 169–94.

Rees, C. (2010) 'Understanding evidence and its utilization in nursing practice,' In K Holland & C. Rees (eds) *Nursing: Evidence -Based Practice Skills*, Oxford: Oxford University Press, pp. 18–38.

Rycroft-Malone, J. (2004) 'The PARIHS framework: a framework for guiding and implementing evidence-based practice', *Journal of Nursing Care Quality*, 19(4): 297–304.

Rycroft-Malone, J. and Bucknall, T. (eds) (2010) *Models and Frameworks for Implementing Evidence-Based Practice: Linking Evidence to Action*, Oxford: Wiley Blackwell.

Schon, D. (1983) *The Reflective Practitioner: How Professionals Think in Action*, New York: Basic Books.

Standing, M. (2011) *Clinical Judgement and Decision Making for Nursing Students*, Exeter: Learning Matters.

Stewart, E. (2006) 'Nursing guidelines: development of catheter care guidelines for Guy's and St Thomas'', *British Journal of Nursing*, 15(8): 420–5.

Thompson, C. (2003) 'Clinical experience as evidence in evidence-based practice', *Journal of Advanced Nursing*, 43(3): 230–7.

Thompson, C. and Dowding, D. (eds) (2009) *Essential Decision Making and Clinical Judgement for Nurses*, Edinburgh: Churchill Livingstone/Elsevier.

Tingle, J. (1990) 'Eusol and the law', *Nursing Times*, 86(12): 70–2.

Xu, W., Towers, A. D., Li, P., and Collett, J. (2006) 'Traditional Chinese medicine in cancer care: perspectives and experiences of patients and professionals in China', *European Journal of Cancer Care*, 15(4): 397–403.

Further Reading

Bullock, I., Clark, J. M., and Rycroft-Malone, J. (eds) (2012) *Adult Nursing Practice: Using Evidence in Care*, Oxford: Oxford University Press.

Thompson, C. (2003) 'Clinical experience as evidence in evidence-based practice', *Journal of Advanced Nursing*, 43(3): 230–7.

Useful Links and Resources

<http://www.joannabriggs.edu.au/Home>

The Joanna Briggs Institute is an Australian-based resource that hosts a wealth of research information. The site offers a wide range of material relating to evidence-based nursing practice that is useful for both nursing practice and education. It offers students an insight into international research studies and links to researchers worldwide who may be undertaking research in the same area of interest. Its Best Practice Guidelines can now be accessed only if a subscribing member.

 <http://global.oup.com/uk/orc/nursing/holland>

The Online Resource Centre for Holland and Rees (2010) offers additional quizzes and links to supplement the material in each chapter. These help students to reflect on their reading and learning, and then allow them to 'test' that learning using the multiple-choice questions and other tests. Tools are also available in some chapters as additional resources, such as those for critiquing an article or an evidence-based PowerPoint presentation.

4

Learning from decision making

Deborah Roberts and Karen Holland

The aims of this chapter are to:

- ➔ explore how and why experiential learning is a useful tool in the development of decision-making skills in nursing;

- ➔ develop the basic skills underpinning reflection;

- ➔ explore how to learn from experience using reflection;

- ➔ learn how to use frameworks for structured reflection and to guide decision-making actions; and

- ➔ consider how experiential learning and reflection contributes to decision making as a qualified nurse.

Introduction

This chapter explores the concept of learning from your experience in clinical practice, and is designed to help you to use reflection as a means of learning both to make decisions in practice and to learn from the decisions that you have made. The use and value of reflective practice will be explored in many of the chapters to come; it is considered to be essential in the development of decision-making skills as a student nurse, and for your ongoing personal and professional development as a qualified registered nurse.

Activity

To ensure that there is a common understanding about some of the terms being used in this chapter (and to avoid duplication of chapter content), you may find it useful to re-read *Chapter 1*. In particular, ensure that you are familiar with terms such as 'critical thinking', 'clinical reasoning', 'clinical judgement', 'intuition', and 'clinical decision making'.

Learning from experience is often referred to as 'experiential learning' and one of its key skills is reflection. In other words, reflection is the key to helping you to use experiences as a student and a person in order to learn from them. This chapter will provide some definitions of reflection and will introduce some commonly used frameworks or models that can help you to develop the underpinning skills required if you are to be a reflective practitioner. There are also activities for you to complete, so that you can begin to use a range of different frameworks that are appropriate to different situations.

To place reflection in the context of your learning to become a nurse and therefore to achieve the appropriate competencies, the Nursing and Midwifery Council (NMC) states that:

> 4. *All nurses must be self-aware and recognize how their own values, principles and assumptions may affect their practice. They must maintain their own personal and professional development, learning from experience, through supervision, feedback, reflection and evaluation.*
>
> (NMC 2010: 20)

We can see from this statement that there appear to be some key assumptions and activities that are seen as working together, including reflection, and these will be explored particularly in this chapter. Reflection on practice, and subsequently for learning from this practice, will be two of the most important aspects that will be addressed. To begin with, however, we need to consider some of the underlying principles in which reflection and reflective practice are embedded.

Experiential learning

Learning from our experiences means that we can either use what we have learned to develop and to enhance future experiences, or alternatively that we can learn from any mistakes that we may have made in the anticipation that we will not make the same ones again.

As a student nurse, you may most commonly do the latter, because most of you are learning new knowledge and skills, and in situations in which there is an opportunity for mistakes to be made.

Making mistakes can be a difficult and uncomfortable experience, and usually there are consequences to our doing so. We need to be careful, however, in how we define 'mistakes', because often these experiences can be considered to be 'errors of judgement', or making wrong or inappropriate decisions.

For example, you might decide not to access academic supervision for one of your assignments, but to go ahead and write an assignment that you think answers the question. However, in doing so, you may misinterpret the brief, with the consequence that your work does not meet the required standard and you are referred, or fail the first attempt, and are required to resubmit.

Mistakes or errors can also occur during your experience in clinical practice, but it is hoped that these will not be mistakes that can endanger the patients in your care, or staff colleagues, or yourself, for most of you learning to engage in or to undertake practice will entail learning a new set of skills that are underpinned by clear rationale and evidence-based knowledge. Many of you will have an opportunity to learn how to learn these skills in the safe environment of what are called 'clinical skills rooms', or 'clinical simulation rooms', in which both the environment and the scenarios around which the skills are taught replicate those that you might find in clinical placements.

In either case, it is important that you take some time to think carefully about how and why you made the mistake, and, most importantly of all, how to ensure that you do not make the same mistake again when a similar situation presents itself.

Reflection is a commonly used term in nursing for this practice of 'thinking carefully about why and how any error' is made, or remembering what and how you did something, and, most importantly, why you did it. It is one way of learning from experience, and of improving your knowledge and skills. However, it is important to stress that learning from experience does not take place only as a result of events that have a negative outcome; it is just as important that nurses are able to identify when things went well, or situations in which the outcome was positive for the nurse and/or the patient, or more widely, for example, when things impact on others or the total care given to the patient. This can help you to ensure that this good practice continues in the future or that it can be the foundation for considering new practice.

Experiential learning can help us to uncover the 'complexities of the clinical world or the classroom or to empower practitioners in either setting, to utilize the invisible and often undervalued knowledge embedded in their practice' (Lumby 1998: 93).

Reflection is not a new idea. Its origins can be traced back to 1933, when John Dewey, an American child psychologist and teacher, defined it as 'Active, persistent and careful consideration of any belief or supposed form of knowledge in the light of the grounds that support it and the further considerations to which it tends' (Dewey 1933: 9).

Reflection is a means by which you can allocate dedicated time to thinking purposefully about clinical and university experiences in order to learn from your experience, and also, most importantly for you as a student nurse, by writing these down in your learning diary.

It is more than simply thinking things over in your mind; we all do this as a matter of course, when we are in the car, going for a walk, at the end of the day, and so on. According to Ruch (2000), learning is a process of reflecting on different sources of knowledge (theoretical, personal, practical, and critical) and incorporates three stages, as follows.

1. Attending to the thoughts and feelings aroused by an event
2. Reassessing the experience in light of its outcomes
3. Experimenting with new approaches in light of the reflection process

Here, Ruch is referring to learning in social work. However, these principles could easily be applied to nursing. More recently in nursing, reflection has been defined as 'Reviewing events from various perspectives' (Bolton 2010) and also 'the process of learning by reviewing what has happened, what could have happened and what may happen in the future through using different approaches' (Rolfe et al. 2011).

We can see from these observations that reflection helps nurses to unpack the sometimes 'messy world' of clinical practice in order to make sense of what took place and, most importantly, to improve personal practice in the future. Often, in nursing, the problems or issues with which nurses are faced are complex and essential decisions are not always easily reached. Experiential learning then involves 'learning by doing'—in other words, it is active, psychomotor, and engaged. You experience something in clinical practice or as part of your university course and then you consider what you would do if a similar situation were to arise again. You might reflect as a mental process—that is, only in your head—or you might write things down in a reflective journal or diary. You can reflect alone or with others (both students and qualified staff). Indeed, you are probably doing this all of the time, but you may not yet recognize that it is reflection.

Consider, for example, an action that you may take in the home: if you make a meal for your family, but things do not quite taste as they did last time, do you revisit the steps that you took? You might even go back and check the recipe, or you might talk with your family about whether or not they found it tasted different and what they thought might be the cause if so.

In terms of learning to be a nurse, you may also be beginning to reflect in the same way. For example, whilst on the way home from working a shift on your placement, do you think about the events of the day? Are there some events that you seem to think about over and over again? Are there some events that seem to be more significant to you than others and to which you return in your thoughts? Do you find yourself thinking about what you will do differently next time? What if the outcome of one of the decisions that you made during the day was the unit manager telling you what a good decision you made and that she was very pleased that you had shown some initiative?

If you have thought about your actions in this way, while also trying to work out alternative actions, then you are already using your experiences to learn through reflection.

The learning is personal to you and concerns developing your self-awareness—in other words, it is personal not public knowledge (although you may share some of your reflections on a clinical practice experience with carefully selected others, such as your personal tutor, or your mentor in clinical practice).

How and why reflection is a useful tool in the development of decision-making skills in nursing

It is important that you recognize that all clinical encounters have the potential to be learning experiences. According to Paul and Heaslip (1995: 40) 'each nurse gains knowledge about nursing practice in such a way that every clinical experience becomes a lesson which informs the next practice experience'. The 'neophyte', or beginning nurse, starts the process by consciously reflecting on his or her knowledge, and by raising questions regarding his or her understanding of what is known and how that knowledge can be applied in the practice situation. The authors qualify this development by asserting that 'The neophyte nurse develops intuitive, skilful performance in practice by reasoning about nursing and applying reflective, critical thought in practice situations, thus gaining greater and greater expert knowledge' (Paul and Heaslip 1995: 41).

As a student nurse, you will have discovered that many practitioners, including your mentors, appear to make decisions without appearing to think about doing them. These 'expert' nurses have learned over time to:

> differentiate the significant data from the insignificant and are able to note what information is missing for safe and effective practice. The expert nurse is able to ask 'What else do I need to know?, Why do I need to know that?, And what difference would this or that fact make to the care of this patient?'
>
> (Paul and Heaslip 1995: 44)

The expert nurse may then appear to act intuitively, but it is not a robotic action—that is, one performed mechanistically—but clearly has thought behind it, given that there is clearly evidence of decisions having been made. This intuitive action in expert practice 'leads to openness to anticipating and recognising deviations from the norm in clinical practice' (Paul and Heaslip 1995: 44).

Activity

Consider one of your placement learning experiences and identify one situation in which it appeared that your mentor or another nurse at the time made decisions without appearing to think about them. Write down what happened, who was there, when it happened, and what was the outcome. If possible, discuss with your mentor how he or she knew what to do, and the knowledge and skills that he or she thought were needed to carry out the activity.

(Continued)

Make a note of your mentor's response (ensuring that you gain his or her permission), and record all of the scenario and notes as part of your reflective diary, which most of you will be required to complete as part of your learning portfolio.

You may now start to consider how this apparently 'seamless' action happens and how you will be able to act like this when you qualify as a nurse. Although we can see clearly that some of the actions relate to clinical reasoning (see **Chapter 1**), the source of others are less clear. We may find some of the answers to these in the work of Donald Schon (1983), in what he called 'reflection in action' and 'reflection on action'.

Reflection in action and reflection on action

Schon (1983), in his seminal work, outlines two types of reflection: 'reflection in action' and 'reflection on action'.

- *Reflection in action* is described as spontaneous, arising when the nurse does not stop to think about his or her actions and decisions, but recognizes a new situation or problem after another and thinks while acting on his or her interpretation of them in a seamless manner.
- *Reflection on action*, as defined by Fitzgerald (1994), is '*the retrospective contemplation of practice in order to uncover the knowledge used in a particular situation, by analysing and interpreting the information recalled*'. In other words, it involves thinking about a (clinical) situation after the event, with the purpose of unpacking what took place and making an interpretation of this analysis.

In terms of reflecting on clinical practice in relation to decision making, three stages are apparent, as follows.

(1) Preparation

Reflective activity starts when students begin to explore what is required of them— referred to by van Manen (1991) as 'anticipatory reflection'—and may be particularly useful for novices. For example, try the following exercise.

....

➕ Exercise

A qualified nurse has asked you to admit a patient or client to the ward; this means that you will have to ask the person a number of questions and fill out the appropriate documentation. You have observed the qualified nurse do this several times before, but now she has asked you to take the lead.

What do you do?

....

You may have decided to use your memory to think about some of the previous occasions on which you have observed an admission of a patient to hospital—thinking carefully about what the nurse did and the manner in which she asked her questions. You may then think about what you are going to say and how you are going to say it. You may even practise saying it to yourself without speaking it out loud. This is what is known as *antici-patory reflection*: you make a plan of action concerning events that are yet to happen.

....

 Top tips

Try to use anticipatory reflection next time you are asked to undertake a relatively new procedure in clinical practice. Try to find some quiet space or time (this might be a physi-cal space, or simply time to stop and think about what you have been asked to do) before you undertake the task. Or make a decision to tell the person who has asked you to undertake the procedure that you either do not want to undertake this, because you are not completely sure of what to do, or, ask them to come with you while you undertake the procedure, in order to ensure that you are doing it correctly. This will be an important decision that you have made, based on your assessment of your own practice skills and knowledge, but also on your reflection on previous experience and practice capabilities.

If you do decide to go ahead and undertake the procedure, try to practise what you will say and how you will say it: you may come up with several versions of the same conversa-tion, based on what the patient or client might say to you.

....

You can even use anticipatory reflection to rehearse psychomotor skills. For example, you may practise your aseptic non-touch technique in the treatment room on the ward or relevant clinical space. You may wish to double check the way in which you will unpack any sterile equipment required, using reflection on previous opportunities or encounters to compare the different patient scenarios.

For further ideas about anticipatory reflection, read Banning, M. (2008) 'A review of clinical decision making: models and current research', *Journal of Clinical Nursing*, 17(2): 187–95.

(2) Engagement in the activity: field experience

Actually being engaged in an activity in which many decisions are required to be made may overwhelm students, because the action in the clinical environment is often fast-paced and observations rapidly follow each other, with insufficient opportunity, if a situation arises that requires immediate decision making, for them to be organized in any structured way.

The clinical learning environment in which you, as a student, are learning to become a nurse can be unstructured, unpredictable, and overwhelming (Papp et al. 2003). Edwards et al. (2004: 249) refer to the work of various authors to develop an overview of the purpose of a planned clinical experience in an appropriate (clinical) placement 'to enable students to develop clinical skills, integrate theory with practice, apply problem solving skills, develop interpersonal skills and become socialized into the formal and informal norms, protocols and expectations of the nursing profession and health care system'.

(3) Processing what has been experienced: making sense of what took place

The idea of processing your experiences and making sense of the event (Boud et al. 1985) means that you have to put both time and effort into reflecting on clinical practice in order to learn from the actual experience. Most importantly, you must try to work out what happened, why you made the decisions that you did, and what was the eventual outcome.

....

 Exercise

In relation to the three stages discussed, try to *make some decisions* about how you intend to find the time and space for regular reflection during your clinical placement. Discuss with your mentor how he or she can help you to make this a reality. It will be a professional development responsibility as part of your nursing course that you ensure that you can use reflection to learn from decision making in practice. Most module timetables in the university include sessions for reflection on practice, during which students have the opportunity to share with their colleagues specific examples of clinical decision making and, through this reflection and sharing, gain possible new insights into their own actions and those of others.

....

Models of reflection: some guidance on their key components

Most models of reflection have some common components, as follows.

(1) Returning to the experience

Within this stage, you are expected to recall the salient events without making any judgements. You should try to describe the event without missing any detail; you may do so by trying to write the incident down or as a mental process. The description may uncover some judgements that were made at the time of the event. This involves the use of memory and, of course, as human beings we recall only what we want to recall.

Further, memory can be flawed. To overcome this, it is a good idea to try to recall the incident soon after the event has taken place, so that events are fresh in your mind. This is particularly relevant when you have been involved in a situation in which you are asked to make a statement to the police.

Consider, for example, a situation in which you made a decision to help a colleague being threatened by a visitor and during which that colleague received a serious injury. In this situation, it would be important for you to record exactly what happened rather than what you *thought* had happened, so documenting your actions as soon as possible after the event would be imperative if it were to be as clear as possible what you saw, what you did, and what others did. Reflecting on the situation later, of course, may cause you to recall some aspects that might have escaped your immediate recall, so making a note of anything else that happened or that you or others did will be as important. An example might be the colour of the assailant's coat or the fact that he or she wore a specific brand of shoes, which you may not have remembered at the time of the incident because everything was happening so quickly.

Writing down what happened for the police must involve recalling clear factual information. When you reflect on a clinical incident, however, there will be the opportunity to consider your feelings, together with why you made the decisions that you made and what evidence was underpinning them, and to make a list of the issues on which you need to find out more information, thereby increasing your knowledge.

(2) Attending to feelings

Within this stage, you will need to use your feelings and, in particular, attend to any negative feelings. It is important to observe the feelings evoked during the experience, because negative feelings about yourself may be a barrier to learning. You might make mistakes and you might feel that, at times, you have made a wrong decision. It is consequently important not to miss this stage out.

 Exercise

Consider the situation of the serious incident in '**(1) Returning to the experience**'. There will definitely be 'feelings' involved in that scenario from your point of view. You may, of course, not have considered them at the time—that is, during your 'reflection in action' phase of the incident. You may, for example, have taken a decision without pausing to consider the outcome of your intervention in order to protect your colleague, but that may have led to a mistake on your part, resulting in an exacerbation of the situation; alternatively, you may have taken a minute or two to consider alternative options, because you had been in a similar situation previously. This 'reflection on action' opportunity may bring back unhappy memories, but also, through this revisiting of prior learning, you can now be more confident in your immediate decision regarding the patient and the threat to your colleague.

It is important to record all of these feelings when undertaking critical reflection on practice and, most importantly, why you had them, and what impact they had on your decision making both at the time and since the situation was resolved.

(3) Re-evaluating the experience

The re-evaluation of an experience may not be completed until the first two stages are completed. This stage involves re-examining the experience in the light of your original intent, associating new knowledge with that which is already possessed, and integrating this knowledge into your conceptual framework. Re-evaluation itself has four stages, which will help you to understand the complete cycle of reflection and reflective practice.

1. *Association*—This stage involves relating new data to that which is already known. How do these new ideas or new knowledge relate to what you already know? How can you begin to bring some of the ideas together?
2. *Integration*—This stage involves seeking relationships among the data. Are there similarities and/or differences between some of the new ideas and things that you already know? Do certain ideas seem to go together?
3. *Validation*—This stage involves determining the authenticity of the resulting ideas and feelings. Am I right to feel this way? Is there evidence that other student nurses have had similar experiences? Here, it is important that you consider your experience in relation to that of other student nurses. You might want to access a nurse education journal that publishes research relating to the experiences of student nurses in clinical placements, such as *Nurse Education Today* and *Nurse Education in Practice* (for example, see Papp et al. 2003).
4. *Appropriation*—This stage involves making this knowledge your own. Indeed, as a student nurse, you may face a difficult struggle to learn some aspects of nursing practice.

For example, Wenger (1998: 47) describes the concept of practice as:

> including both the explicit and the tacit. It includes what is said and what is left unsaid, what is represented and what is assumed, subtle cues, untold rules of thumb; most of which may never be articulated, yet they are unmistakable signs of membership of the community of practice.

In nursing in particular, there may be many unwritten, implicit rules for you, as a student, to overcome. Reflection is one way of thinking about some of those unwritten rules in order to make sense of clinical practice, and to make appropriate decisions in relation to patient care and your own nursing actions.

Case study 4.1 Student reflection on an experience in clinical placement

Having settled into the department and familiarized myself with the routine, it was possible for me to contribute as a member of the team, taking on some of the responsibilities and roles.

There was a call on the 'standby' phone in the accident and emergency (A&E) department, which stated that a 76-year-old male had been found collapsed on a nearby street by the ambulance crew; he wasn't breathing and there was no sign of a pulse, and so they had started cardio-pulmonary resuscitation (CPR). It would take them 6 minutes to reach the department. The staff who were allocated by the coordinator to be in the resuscitation room started to get their individual equipment ready for the patient's arrival. I stood there and watched in amazement at their efficiency. I could feel my heart pumping faster and I wondered how long the ambulance would be. Those 6 minutes felt like 6 seconds. When the ambulance pulled up outside the department, my mentor, Jane, ran out to meet the paramedics. I followed, not knowing what else to do. The doors opened for me to see an elderly gentleman lying on a stretcher with blood covering his face and chest. It was a shock to see. Jane took over from the paramedics and started CPR. The paramedics pulled the patient into the resuscitation room on the trolley; I ran behind them with adrenaline pumping round my body, wondering what the next step was. This was a new experience for me.

The team was waiting for the patient. It started to get noisy in the cubicle: the team leader was phoning for X-rays and electrocardiograms (ECGs); others were trying to find any identification that would tell us who the gentleman was. The patient was still not breathing and had no pulse; the team leader told me to commence chest compressions. Pressing down firmly and smoothly, I did the compressions. These should be done at a rate of about 80 per minute. I paused while the team leader gave the oxygen and I restarted the compressions, both of us working in a rhythm. I was amazed at the depth of concentration I had on the patient, watching his chest rise and fall with the oxygen being pushed into his lungs by the team leader. I was hoping for some signs of life.

My arms were starting to ache, and I could feel the heat from the overhead light beginning to make me sweat and feel hot. I looked up to see the time: I'd been doing my compressions for nearly ten minutes. I thought of having a break. I looked around for someone to take over: there was nobody free. They were all busy carrying out their own tasks for the patient. I could carry on—I wasn't exhausted—but I just felt, at the time, that I needed a rest. I did wonder how long the team were going to keep on trying and who out of the team would disengage the procedures. It was then that the circulation nurse asked if I was alright. I said 'yes', straight away, without even thinking, because I didn't want the rest of the team to think I wasn't strong enough mentally or physically. I carried on, trying to be professional. The clock was showing 1.20 p.m.: I'd been doing CPR for twenty minutes. I was hot and sweaty; my arms ached like mad; I'd started to get cramp in my calves: I was exhausted. I wanted to stop now—but I didn't want to ask. Just then, the team leader asked the team if anyone in the room felt that the procedure should continue. I could hear the team discuss the outcome, which they all felt should be to discontinue treatment. The team leader thanked everyone for doing their best and asked me

(Continued)

Case study 4.1 (Continued)

to step down. My legs were shaking as I stepped down from the bed, and my arms and neck were so stiff. Physically, I withdrew from the situation—but not mentally. I looked and looked at the patient with sadness, because now it was final: now, he was dead; before, there had been hope.

I sat down on a chair and watched the team leave the room. Reflecting then, I was thinking more about his family, knowing that, while I knew he was dead, they didn't. I wondered where he was going when he collapsed in the street . . .

Question

Can you identify any of the elements of reflection already discussed in this chapter within this account of one student's experience on placement in an A&E department?

The incident in **Case study 4.1** could be referred to as a *critical incident*, or a *significant event*—a term that will be familiar to many of you, because it is used to refer to what students have to describe and then critically reflect upon in order to demonstrate practice learning or for a theoretical nursing assignment. (See Gimenez 2011 for guidance on how to write such an assignment.)

The event was clearly significant for this student and this is evident in the way in which the student is able to articulate what took place: there is a depth and detail to the description. We really get a sense of what it was like for the student physically and mentally during this resuscitation event. You will also experience significant events of this kind and, to enable you to learn as much as possible from them, try to write about them after the event in as much detail as possible. Do not forget that a significant event does not have to be a negative experience and, for the student in **Case study 4.1**, it can be seen clearly as a learning experience that generated positive and negative thoughts—although we can be sure that, when the student discussed this with his or her personal tutor or wrote up the second part of the reflection, which would focus on the actual learning from the experience, there would be many issues arising that we can, in reading it, only begin to recognize.

Activity

Read through *Case study 4.1* again and make notes on the major issues that you think this student learned about the decision-making situations described within. Consider those made by the student and those made by other members of the

(Continued)

> multidisciplinary team (MDT). How did the scenario also demonstrate how this student had made links between theoretical knowledge, such as the underpinning physiological knowledge used, and the decisions made? One example could be that the observation of 'no pulse and not breathing' led to the decision to undertake cardio-pulmonary resuscitation.

The following section of the chapter provides a brief overview of some commonly used frameworks or models of reflection that you can use to undertake your own reflection on practice in relation to decision making, which is the focus of this book. Frameworks or models can be useful in helping you to learn from decision making because they provide a structure for your thinking and your reflective writing. Some people find a structure to be useful; others will find them restrictive and prefer simply to write their ideas down as free text. You might find it useful, when you are starting to think about the development of your own decision-making skills, to start by using frameworks or models to guide you.

Activity

Read *Case study 4.1* again. Do you think that the student actually used a model of reflection to describe the scenario and his or her own feelings during and after the event?

Frameworks or models of reflection

Boud et al.'s model of reflection

Boud et al.'s (1985) model of reflection includes most of the elements that have just been described. The first step in the process begins with the experience itself. This may have had an impact on you in terms of how you feel about your own actions or those of someone else, or you might be unsure of your feelings about an event. Alternatively, the event itself may provoke other ideas that you need to explore. The second step is concerned with the process of reflection; the final step is concerned with adopting a new behaviour or skill. Within this last stage, you will consider how you will use your newfound knowledge, skills, or attitudes towards the event or similar issues.

These steps can be expressed as follows.

1. *Experiences*—This step is concerned with behaviour, ideas or feelings
2. *Reflective processes*—These processes involve:
   - returning to the experience (think about the event in terms of what happened and relive the situation in your mind, focusing on all of your senses—what you saw, heard, smelled, and felt);

- attending to feelings (this can be more difficult than it sounds, because there may be uncomfortable feelings that you need to acknowledge); and
- re-evaluating the experience (putting things into context, because your original thoughts about an event may not be the same as they are now).

3. *Outcomes of reflection*—These can involve:
   - clarification of an issue (this involves really focusing on what the issue is or was);
   - a new way of behaving or of doing something (as a result of the activity and as a result of thinking about it in this purposive way, you may decide to undertake some reading to bridge knowledge gaps or to develop new perspectives on the situation);
   - the development of a skill (you may have to develop new techniques);
   - the resolution of a problem (as a result of this activity, you may find that the initial uncomfortable feelings have subsided and that you now feel differently; you may have gained new knowledge and skills, which means that if a similar situation were to arise again, you would respond differently, from a more knowledgeable evidence base); and
   - greater confidence in what you are doing or modified priorities.

Gibbs' model of reflection

Gibbs' (1998) reflective cycle (see **Figure 4.1**) is relatively easy to use, because the stages of the model are clearly explained. Many universities in the United Kingdom

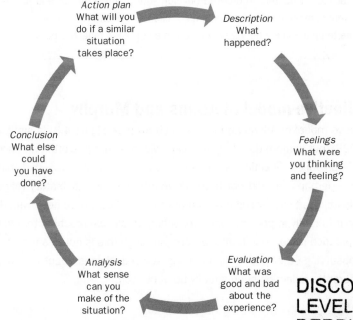

Figure 4.1 Gibbs' model of reflection: the reflective cycle.
Source: Gibbs (1998).

have adopted this model for their curriculums and for student use when writing about experiences in clinical practice. The model asks you to develop a clear and detailed description of the situation. However, as you progress through the course or take on further postgraduate study and begin writing at higher academic levels, critical analysis should be visible at each stage of the process, not only in the sections labelled as such.

....

 Exercise

Try to think of a situation in clinical practice in which you have been involved in which you communicated with a patient, a member of staff, or a patient's relative. Try to think of a situation in which you feel that you used good communication skills (these might be verbal, non-verbal, or a mixture of the two).

Use Gibbs' reflective framework to structure your thoughts and write down some ideas relating to each section of the model, paying particular attention to a description of the event and your feelings at the time.

For the evaluation section, try to identify why the event went well: what did you do or say that made this a positive event? If you can, try to think about some of the theories of communication of which you are aware and make a note of these as well. This will help you to start to apply theories to practice situations as in evidence-based practice (see **Chapter 3**); this is a skill that you will find useful for your future clinical encounters, but also when you undertake your academic assignments, which will often require you to demonstrate an ability to do this. This is often described as using 'critical reflection'.

Finally, try to write down some ideas concerning how you will use this knowledge in your future practice encounters in order to develop your practice further and to ensure that more of your communication with patients or clients is positive.

Use the template in **Figure 4.2** to write down all of these reflective activities.

....

The reflective model of Atkins and Murphy

The reflective model of Atkins and Murphy (1994) (see **Figure 4.3**) is similar to that of Gibbs (1998), but is more detailed and acknowledges that it is often an uncomfortable feeling that provokes reflection on practice. You may feel, at times, that things did not go to plan—perhaps you did not have an opportunity for anticipatory reflection—and that events have left you feeling awkward or that you should have dealt with the incident differently. It is really important, when reflecting on clinical practice, that you focus on your own practice rather than that of others. Although this is not to say that you will not learn by observing other people and making some decisions about how you would do things differently, reflection should really be about *you*.

Description	
Feelings	
Evaluation	
Analysis	
Conclusion	
Action plan	

Figure 4.2 Template for Gibbs' reflective cycle.
Source: Gibbs (1998).

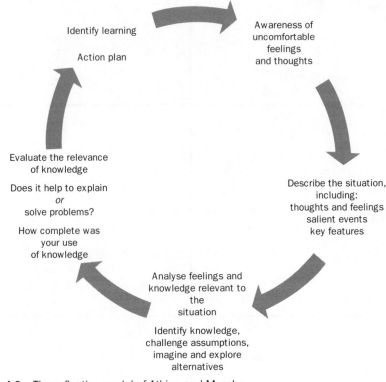

Figure 4.3 The reflective model of Atkins and Murphy.
Source: Atkins and Murphy (1994).

⊕ **Exercise**

Try to think about an event during which your communication skills were not as good as they could have been. Use the headings of the Atkins and Murphy (1994) model to write down your thoughts, paying particular attention to your description of the event and your feelings. Just as in the last exercise, try to introduce some theory or ideas that you have read about; this will help you to understand what took place.

You can use the template in **Figure 4.4** to write down your thoughts and feelings.

Johns' model for structured reflection

Johns' (2004) model for structured reflection can be used as a guide for analysis of a critical incident (significant event) or general reflection on an experience. It is much more structured than the models of Gibbs (1998) or Atkins and Murphy (1994), but it too outlines a set number of stages that comprise the reflection cycle.

Awareness of uncomfortable feelings or thoughts	
Description of the event	
Analysis	
Evaluation	
Learning plan	

Figure 4.4 Template for Atkins and Murphy's reflective cycle.
Source: Atkins and Murphy (1994).

The five stages of Johns' model are as follows.

1. *'Bringing the mind home'*—This emphasizes the importance of finding a physical or virtual space in which experiential learning can take place.
2. *Description*—Write a description of the experience and ask: 'What are the key issues within this description to which I need to pay attention?' Your description here should be about the facts (not your feelings), although it takes practice to separate these out. The key issues should be what makes you feel uncomfortable or elements of the situation that you did not understand.

3. *Reflection on what occurred*—This will include asking yourself the following questions.
   - 'How was I feeling and what made me feel that way?'
   - 'What was I trying to achieve? Did I respond effectively?'
   - 'What were the consequences of my actions for the patient, others, and myself?'
   - 'How were others feeling and what made them feel that way?'
   - 'What factors influenced the way I was feeling, thinking, or responding?'
   - 'What knowledge might have informed me?'
   - 'To what extent did I act for the best and in tune with my values?'

   This section is where your feelings should come to the forefront of your description or analysis. When you start to discuss the consequences for your actions, you should start to introduce the literature here to begin to support your actions or to help to explain what was going on—that is, you should offer evidence to support your actions and/or decision making. The influencing factors should also be where you begin to bring in the literature, so that your reflections are evidence-based. However, you may also discuss personal factors, including your own beliefs and values.

4. *Alternatives*—This stage involves considering the following.
   - 'How does this situation connect with previous experiences?'
   - 'How might I respond more effectively if I were to be confronted with this situation again?'
   - 'What would be the consequences of alternative actions for the patient, others, and myself?'

   This section prepares you for future action and some say that it is the most important element of reflective practice: deciding to do it better or differently next time. The other choices should be firmly rooted in the literature, again to ensure that your future actions are evidence-based.

5. *Changes*—You will consider the following questions.
   - 'How do I feel about this experience *now*?'
   - 'Am I now more able to support myself and others better as a consequence?'

   This section goes back to considering your views about nursing practice. Now that you have read the literature and perhaps found some explanations for either your own actions or the situation itself, what do you think now?

....

➕ Exercise

Try to use the headings from Johns' model to structure your thoughts in relation to a recent clinical incident (significant event). Try to think of an incident that you consider to be significant; this might be either a positive or negative experience. An example of a positive experience could be teaching a patient to give his or her own insulin injection and receiving positive feedback from your mentor. An example of a negative experience could be a situation in which the staff in your placement refer to you only as 'the student' for the whole of your four-week placement.

Learning to reflect: using a model of your choice

Once you have completed this last exercise, using a specific model, you now need to consider all of the models and frameworks that have been used in this chapter, and to undertake a focused activity related to your own field of practice. First, we return to **Case study 4.1**, which you can use as a guide to writing your own reflection on a situation and a critical review of your decision-making activities in that field-specific practice situation.

 Exercise

Having used a range of models, make a decision about which one(s) you found most useful in reflecting on your practice learning experience generally and for a specific situation, and which you might want to use again in future.

Return to **Case study 4.1**, in which a student nurse helped to resuscitate a patient in A&E.

- Try to use one of the models to restructure the account. Can you identify different sections within the reflection?
- Put yourself in the position of the student and think about what you would have done, or would do, if you were ever in a similar situation.
- What factors do you think you would take into consideration in your decision making?

In your response to this part of the exercise, you may consider the anticipatory reflection that begins when the 'standby' (emergency room) phone rings. What sorts of decision are required here in order to prepare for the arrival of the patient and in order to prepare yourself for what is about to take place?

You might want to think about the knowledge base that underpins CPR, and how many compressions per minute are required and what the ratio of breaths to compressions is.

- Would you decide to undertake the compressions, like the student in the case study, or would you take another decision: to refuse, perhaps?
- Would you decide to ask for a break once you got tired? How long would you undertake resuscitation before asking such a question?
- How do you think you would feel if the resuscitation attempt were stopped?
- What are the ethical and moral implications of having information of which the patient's loved ones are not aware? How would this make you feel?

Finally, you might decide to use an alternative framework to write up your interpretation of events or your own experience (see **Figure 4.5**).

Description of the event	
Who was there?	
What happened?	
How did I feel?	
What have I learned?	
Do you want to talk about this with someone else? If so, who?	
Decisions regarding future practice	

Figure 4.5 A general framework for use in a structured reflection.

As you progress through your pre-registration programme, you will find your own ways of using your experiences to make decisions. **Part 3** of this book includes many examples of newly qualified nurses across all of the fields of practice reflecting on their own decision-making skills in action.

Conclusion

This chapter has provided you with an overview of the principles of learning from experience and reflection, and has introduced you to some frameworks or models that can be used to help you to make sense of clinical encounters and, in particular, those decision-making activities. Like all skills in nursing, reflection takes practice. In other words, it will require time and effort on your part in order to learn from your experiences. You can reflect on your own or with others, but the most important thing about reflection is that you commit to making future actions better, based on what you have learned from the event. Reflecting can also help you to refine your decision-making skills, and the use of reflection will be evident in the following chapters.

References

Atkins, S. and Murphy, K. (1994) 'Reflective practice', *Nursing Standard*, 8(39): 49–54.

Banning, M. (2008) 'A review of clinical decision making: models and current research', *Journal of Clinical Nursing*, 17(2): 187–95.

Bolton, G. (2010) *Reflective Practice: Writing and Professional Development*, 3rd edn, London: Sage.

Boud, D., Keogh, R., and Walker, D. (eds) (1985) *Reflection: Turning Experience into Learning*, New York: Routledge Falmer.

Carper, B. (1978) 'Fundamental patterns of knowing', *Advances in Nursing Science*, 1(1): 13–23.

Dewey, J. (1933) *How We Think*, New York: Heath.

Edwards, H., Smith, S., Courtney, M., Finlayson, K., and Chapman, H. (2004) 'The impact of clinical placement location on nursing students' competence and preparedness for practice', *Nurse Education Today*, 24(4): 248–55.

Fitzgerald, M. (1994) 'Theories of reflection for learning', in A. Palmer, S. Burns, and C. Bulman (eds) *Reflective Practice in Nursing: The Growth of the Professional Practitioner*, Oxford: Blackwell, pp. 63–84.

Gibbs, G. (1998) *Learning by Doing: A Guide to Teaching and Learning Methods*, Oxford: Oxford Further Education Unit.

Gimenez, J. (2011) *Writing for Nursing and Midwifery Students*, 2nd edn, Basingstoke: Palgrave Macmillan.

Johns, C. (2004) *Becoming a Reflective Practitioner: A Reflective and Holistic Approach to Clinical Nursing, Practice Development and Clinical Supervision*, London: Blackwell.

Lumby, J. (1998) 'Transforming nursing through reflective practice', in C. Johns and D. Freshwater (eds) *Transforming Nursing through Reflective Practice*, Oxford: Blackwell Science, pp. 91–103.

Nursing and Midwifery Council (2010) *Standards for Pre-Registration Nursing Education*, London: NMC.

Papp, I., Markkanen, M., and von Bonsdorff, M. (2003) 'Clinical environment as a learning environment: student nurses' perceptions concerning clinical learning experiences', *Nurse Education Today*, 23(4): 262–8.

Paul, R. and Heaslip, P. (1995) 'Critical thinking and intuitive nursing practice', *Journal of Advanced Nursing*, 22(7): 40–7.

Rolfe, G., Jasper, M., and Freshwater, D. (2011) *Critical Reflection in Practice: Generating Knowledge for Care*, 2nd edn, Basingstoke: Palgrave Macmillan.

Ruch, G. (2000) 'Self and social work: towards an integrated model of learning', *Journal of Social Work Practice*, 14(2): 99–112.

Schon, D. A. (1983) *The Reflective Practitioner*, London: Temple Smith.

Schon, D. A. (1987) *Educating the Reflective Practitioner: How Professionals Think in Action*, San Francisco, CA: Jossey-Bass.

van Manen, M. (1991) *The Tact of Teaching*, New York: New York Press.

Webb, L. (ed.) (2011) *Nursing: Communication Skills in Practice*, Oxford: Oxford University Press.

Wenger, E. (1998) *Communities of Practice: Learning, Meaning and Identity*, Cambridge: Cambridge University Press.

Further Reading

Daly, W. M. (1998) 'Critical thinking as an outcome of nursing education: what is it? Why is it important to nursing practice?', *Journal of Advanced Nursing*, 28(2): 323–31.

Price, B. and Harrington, A. (2010) *Critical Thinking and Writing for Students*, Exeter: Learning Matters Ltd.

Timmins, F. (2008) *Making Sense of Portfolios*, Maidenhead: Open University Press.

Webb, L. (ed.) (2011) *Nursing: Communication Skills in Practice*, Oxford: Oxford University Press.

Useful Links and Resources

 <http://global.oup.com/uk/orc/nursing/webb/>

The Online Resource Centre that accompanies ch. 15 of Webb 2011.See especially 'Reflective Practice: The Frameworks'.

<http://www.science.ulster.ac.uk/nursing/mentorship/docs/learning/reflectiononpractice.pdf>

A guide entitled *Reflection on Practice*, from the Making Practice-Based Learning Work project led by University of Ulster.

<http://www.science.ulster.ac.uk/nursing/mentorship/docs/learning/RoyalBromptonV3.pdf>

A practical guide entitled *Learning and Assessing through Reflection*, from the Making Practice-Based Learning Work project led by University of Ulster.

Decision making and achieving competence

PART 2

This part of the book will explore the use of decision making in achieving competence to practise within the four Nursing and Midwifery Council (NMC) domains. It will offer real-life case studies to illustrate key issues and how the student can learn to make effective decisions in his or her journey to becoming a qualified nurse. These chapters are applicable to student nurses pursuing all fields of practice or pathways in this journey. In many of the competencies, the use of decision-making knowledge and skills is implied rather than made explicit. Some of them, however, are more visible and direct. Given that nursing practice is such a complex activity, we know that decision making will take place in a variety of ways, including when giving direct care, when working with service users and carers, and when working alongside others in the multidisciplinary team (MDT).

5

Professional values and decision making

Ruth Chadwick

The aims of this chapter are to:

- ➔ explore the use of decision making in relation to professional values in nursing;

- ➔ explore how decision making impacts on the professional values to achieve competence to practise as a nurse;

- ➔ demonstrate through case studies how different decisions impact on the student nurse's journey to becoming a qualified registered nurse; and

- ➔ demonstrate the role that the Nursing and Midwifery Council has in relation to the student nurse and achieving professional values competencies.

Introduction

This is the first chapter in the part of the book exploring each of the four domains comprising the Nursing and Midwifery Council (NMC) *Standards for Pre-Registration Nursing Education* (NMC 2010) in which the student nurse in the United Kingdom has to demonstrate attainment of the specific competencies to achieve registration as a nurse. In keeping with the overall aims of the book, the aim of this chapter is to help you to develop your decision-making skills in the domain of 'professional values'. It will offer real-life case studies to illustrate key issues and how you, as a student, can learn to make effective decisions in your journey to becoming a registered nurse.

Because this book is written by registered nurses, many of whom work in education, you will probably not be very surprised to learn that we think your decision to become a nurse could be one of the best decisions that you have made to date—but do you really understand what lies before you? Before you begin to be concerned about the 'right-ness' of your decision to become a nurse, it is important to remember that there are many individuals who are there to help you on your professional journey, including your personal tutors, mentors and other practitioners in practice, lecturers, other students, and most importantly the patients and clients for whom you will be caring and with whom you will be working. In addition, you will have friends and family who offer a different kind of support to you, as well as those organizations that can offer professional support to you as a student nurse and subsequently to you as a qualified nurse.

This chapter also intends to help you to appreciate the significance of the NMC's *Guidance on Professional Conduct for Nursing and Midwifery Students* (NMC 2011) as you embark on your professional and personal journey to become a registered practitioner who is able to demonstrate the required standards of conduct, performance, and ethics, as expressed in *The Code: Standards of Conduct, Performance and Ethics for Nurses and Midwives* (NMC 2008).

Safeguarding the public, and ensuring professional values and integrity

Safeguarding the public is one of the essential requirements of professional practice in nursing. We can see this in the generic competence that must be achieved by all student nurses across all four fields of practice in that, in addition to safeguarding the public, it also focuses on the professional values and integrity to which nurses must adhere (see **Box 5.1**).

Decision making, however, in relation to personal and professional values, extends beyond the competencies required by the NMC. In order to make and take effective decisions in nursing practice, individuals should first consider their own personal and professional beliefs and values, and how these might impact on their clinical decision making.

Box 5.1 Nursing and Midwifery Council competencies for entry to the register

Domain 1: Professional values

Generic standard for competence

All nurses must act first and foremost to care for and safeguard the public. They must practise autonomously and be responsible and accountable for safe, compassionate, person-centred, evidence-based nursing that respects and maintains dignity and human rights. They must show professionalism and integrity and work within recognized professional, ethical and legal frameworks. They must work in partnership with other health and social care professionals and agencies, service users, their carers and families in all settings, including the community, ensuring that decisions about care are shared.

(NMC 2010: 13)

All of us are members of the public who may require nursing care at some point in our lives and, as such, it could be argued that we all have a vested interest in ensuring that we both know about and also uphold the values and standards of the nursing profession.

Deciding to become a nurse is a big decision to make (see **Chapter 2**). Patients and the public truly value the work that you will be doing, and you will need to learn about the behaviour and conduct that the public and the profession expect of you as a student nurse.

The public does not always see the difference between student nurses and registered nurses, which is one of the reasons why the NMC Guidance is so important and why it is also essential that you understand what is expected of you as a student nurse who is preparing to become a qualified nurse.

In the UK, nursing is a regulated profession and its regulatory body is the NMC. In order to practise in the UK, all nurses, midwives, and health visitors must be currently registered with the NMC. This involves adhering to the Standards that are set by this professional body and upholding the professional Code. It also means, in common with all health care regulatory bodies, paying a fee to maintain your registration. However, this last issue may not be a priority consideration for you at the start of your journey to becoming a nurse.

The Nursing and Midwifery Council

The NMC in the UK exists, in the main, to safeguard the health and well-being of the public, as do similar organizations in other parts of the world. It does this by making sure that the public are cared for only by nurses who are entitled and deemed fit (in terms of their 'fitness to practise' as nurses) to be on the register. The NMC has a web page that is specifically aimed at members of the general public and allows them to read what it is that the Council does, what it is for, and how it safeguards the health and well-being of the general public: **<http://www.nmc-uk.org/General-public/>**

The NMC works with higher education institutions to make sure that programmes of study for student nurses are of an appropriate standard both in the university and clinical settings. These standards can be found online at: **<http://www.nmc-uk.org/ Educators/Standards-for-education/>**

The NMC also is a source of advice and guidance for registered practitioners whether they are working in clinical practice, management, research, or education. You will hear many references to the NMC and even more about The Code (NMC 2008) during your pre-registration programme. The Code is the foundation of good nursing and midwifery practice; all qualified nurses and midwives have to follow it. The Code is a key tool in safeguarding the health and well-being of the public, and you need to be familiar with it. **Box 5.2** outlines the four basic principles on which The Code is based.

> ### Box 5.2 The Code: Standards of Conduct, Performance, and Ethics for Nurses and Midwives
>
> **The people in your care must be able to trust you with their health and wellbeing**
> **To justify that trust, you must:**
> - *make the care of people your first concern, treating them as individuals and respecting their dignity*
> - *work with others to protect and promote the health and wellbeing of those in your care, their families and carers, and the wider community*
> - *provide a high standard of practice and care at all times*
> - *be open and honest, act with integrity and uphold the reputation of your profession.*
>
> (NMC 2008: 2)

Your conduct as a nursing or midwifery student is based on the four core principles set out in The Code. The Student Guidance (NMC 2011) sets out the personal and professional conduct expected of you as a nursing student in order for you to be fit to practise as a registered nurse. This Guidance is based on the strict standards set out in The Code, and is designed to help you to understand and uphold similar high standards while you are learning, and to make sure that you are fit to practise when the time comes for you to graduate and qualify. You will be working towards these standards during your pre-registration programme.

Activity

Obtain a copy of and read *The Code* (NMC 2008) and the *Guidance on Professional Conduct for Nursing and Midwifery Students* (NMC 2011). Compare them and identify some of the essential differences in relation to 'professional accountability' and what you need to be 'fit to practise'.

Being fit to practise as a nurse

During your pre-registration programme, you will develop the knowledge, skills, and attitudes that you need to be a registered nurse and therefore to be 'fit to practise'.

Being fit to practise also means *having good health* and *good character* throughout your pre-registration programme, to undertake your learning to become a nurse safely and effectively as a student.

- *Good health* is necessary to undertake practice as a nurse or a midwife. It means that a person must be capable of safe and effective practice without supervision.
- *Good character* is also important, because it is expected that nurses and midwives must be honest and trustworthy. Your good character as a student nurse will be assessed on the basis of your conduct, behaviour, and attitude, and in terms of how you demonstrate this during both your placement learning and that in the university.

It is important to note that a person's character must be sufficiently good for him or her to be capable of safe and effective practice without supervision. Of course, there are always going to be questions as to the meaning of 'sufficiently good', and there are problems in determining and interpreting the term in a consistent and fair manner.

The NMC emphasizes the importance of negative consideration of past conduct 'not considered compatible with professional registration' and its Guidance makes clear the centrality of past actions as potentially negative in its assessments of good character. We will return to some of these in the case studies focused on decision making.

Your education institution will have made an assessment of your character at the time that you applied to pursue a pre-registration programme in nursing. Good character is important, and The Code emphasizes honesty and trustworthiness as key values for both nurses and midwives (NMC 2008).

To qualify as a nurse and to be included on the NMC register, all student nurses have to be assessed throughout their three-year programme of study. They will also have to be assessed at key points during those three years as a compulsory requirement of the NMC. These key points are called 'progression points'; the first of these takes place at the end of the first year (See Table 5.1 for an example).

Activity

Look at all of the competencies related to 'Professional values' and 'Ensuring safety of people' only in *Table 5.1*. Determine what kinds of decisions you can make to demonstrate that you have met these competencies to progress to the second year of your programme. (Please note that these will be assessed in practice by your mentors and that you may also have assessments that you have to pass to achieve academic credits alongside those in practice.) Focus in particular on those related to 'Safety and safeguarding people of all ages'.

Box 5.3 First progression point criteria

Criteria that must be met as a minimum requirement by progression point one in any practice setting where people are receiving care, or through simulation.

Table 5.1 Examples of first progression point criteria relating to professional values

Areas associated with safety and safeguarding people of all ages, their carers and their families		Related competency domain
...	...	...
6	Is able to recognize, and work within, the limitations of their own knowledge and skills and professional boundaries, understanding that they are responsible for their own actions.	Professional values ...
...	...	...
15	Acts in a manner that is attentive, kind, sensitive, compassionate and non-discriminatory, that values diversity and acts within professional boundaries.	Professional values ...
16	Understands the principles of confidentiality and data protection. Treats information as confidential, except where sharing is required to safeguard and protect people.	Professional values ...
17	Practises honestly and with integrity, applying the principles of *The code: Standards of conduct, performance and ethics for nurses and midwives* (2008) and the *Guidance on professional conduct for nursing and midwifery students* (2009).	Professional values ...
18	Acts in a way that values the roles and responsibilities of others in the team and interacts appropriately.	Professional values ...

Source: NMC (2010: Annexe 2)

During your pre-registration programme, you will learn about the behaviour and conduct that the public expects of a nurse, but, as the NMC notes, 'it is important that, even as a student, you conduct yourself professionally at all times in order to justify the trust the public places in our professions' (NMC 2011).

All education providers are expected by the NMC to include the student Guidance in the content of their pre-registration programmes and to use it to determine a student's fitness to practise. If there are ever concerns about your fitness to practise, these will be investigated and addressed by your university or education provider, often in partnership with the National Health Service (NHS) or other health and social care organization in which you have been undertaking a placement learning experience. The NMC investigates all allegations made against nurses and midwives questioning their fitness to practise, including allegations of misconduct, lack of competence, and ill health. The

Council's main purpose in doing this is to safeguard the health and well-being of the public. (We will be returning to some of these later in the chapter when looking at decisions that some nurses have made.)

When you have successfully completed your programme, your university will inform the NMC that you have met the education and practice standards, and are of good health and good character. If you are deemed fit to practise, you will then be eligible to apply to join the register, for which you will have to pay a fee, as provided for by the Nursing and Midwifery Council (Fees) Rules 2004 (see **<http://www.nmc-uk.org/ Documents/Legislation/Fees-Rules-2004-Consolidated-text-2011.pdf>** for an amended version dated November 2011).

··

➡ Top Tips

It is important that you are aware that your behaviour and conduct, both during your programme and in your personal life, may have an impact on your fitness to practise. Scrutiny of your behaviour and conduct began during your recruitment and selection, and continued through pre-induction, registration, and induction, and will continue throughout the programme. How you conduct yourself in the real or virtual world at all times matters, and it is imperative that you remember that this applies to your personal life just as much as it does as your professional life. How you behave at 3 a.m. on a Sunday following an evening out celebrating a birthday may significantly impact upon your fitness to practise at work at 7 a.m. on a Monday. It may even compromise your ability to complete your programme of studies, and jeopardize your prospect of becoming and remaining a registered nurse.

··

It is important that you understand the Guidance, and how it will impact on many decisions that you make in both your personal and professional life. Discuss it with your peers and your personal tutors, and think carefully about how and when it might apply in everyday settings. Reading this chapter will provide you with some helpful pointers to do this.

Professional values and decision making as a student nurse

We can now begin to consider all of this information on the issue of professional values, safeguarding the public, and personal and professional behaviour in the context of decision making by you as a student nurse.

Activity

Either on your own or in discussion with a group of your peers, consider how a student nurse should behave while in the university and in clinical practice with respect to the four core principles of The Code (NMC 2008). To remind you, these are:

- *make the care of people your first concern, treating them as individuals and respecting their dignity*
- *work with others to protect and promote the health and wellbeing of those in your care, their families and carers, and the wider community*
- *provide a high standard of practice and care at all times*
- *be open and honest, act with integrity and uphold the reputation of your profession.*

(NMC 2008: 2)

Compile a list of expected behaviours, either on your own or within your group. Share your thoughts with other individuals or with other groups. Are there similarities or differences between them?

To help you with your answers, refer to your own university guidance on good practice for student nurses, and also access and re-read The Code (NMC 2008) and student Guidance (NMC 2011) again.

 Top Tips

The Code and the Guidance

- Read it!
- Keep it!
- Follow it!

Applying The Code to the use of social networking sites

You may be relieved to know that the NMC is not opposed to student and registered nurses and midwives using social networking sites. In fact, the NMC itself makes use of both Facebook and Twitter. However, to ensure that you use these sites safely and wisely, the NMC has published some useful guidance in relation to using social networking sites, available online at **<http://www.nmc-uk.org/Nurses-and-midwives/Advice-by-topic/A/Advice/Social-networking-sites/>**

Activity

Visit the web page and consider whether you are complying with the NMC's principles in relation to the use of social networking sites.

Find out exactly what your university's guidance is on the use of these sites for communicating between each other on all aspects of your course of study.

Having read neither this guidance, nor The Code, on social networking sites will not be helpful if you are found not to have complied with that guidance.

As an example, consider **Case study 5.1**.

Case study 5.1 Sharing views through social media: a cautionary tale

A student, unhappy with the way in which a lecturer delivered one of the teaching sessions in the university, posted a very derogatory review of the session on her Facebook site, including the lecturer's name, which university it was, and which course she was undertaking, as well as what she thought personally about this lecturer. The outcome was that a colleague of the lecturer became aware of this public-facing message and escalated the incident to become a disciplinary matter, in which the student nurse's 'fitness to practise' as a nurse was called into question. Her decision to write such a comment because she was angry about the session and the lecturer's teaching was no excuse, because there are formal mechanisms in most universities, such as a staff–student committee, that she might have used to explore these kinds of issues. In this case, the student decided for herself that she did not want to be a nurse because of all of the 'stupid rules' and she chose to leave the course before any disciplinary action could be taken.

Questions

1. What are the privacy settings for your social networking sites?
2. Have you ever decided to accept someone on a social networking site who you did not know personally as a friend?
3. Are your friends real or virtual?

Top Tips

- Remember that *everything* you post online is in the public arena.
  - It will *always* be there.
  - It will be shared and you will not retain control over the information.
- Think before you post and share your personal information (or make comments about others).
- Do not drink alcohol and post online at the same time.
- Keep your personal life and professional life separate.
- Consider using different modes of social networking for different aspects of your life.
- Think carefully before accepting social networking invitations, and remember that you can reject requests and block individuals or delete 'friends'.
- If you tell people in an online environment that you are a student nurse, you must always uphold the standards set by the regulatory body, so that you do not present a tarnished image of the profession.
- Do not use social networks to keep in touch with current or past clients.
- Do not ever discuss work- or patient/client-related matters online, even anonymously.
- Do make full use of privacy settings.
- Maintain confidentiality at all times.
- Never post photographs of clients. In fact, you should never take photographs of clients.
- Never use social networks or the Internet for illegal activities.

There have been a handful of cases before the NMC's 'fitness to practise' (FTP) panels that involved the use of social networking sites or other Internet-based activity. In most of these cases, use of the Internet has been only a small part of the overall case. Full information on the types of case that come before the FTP panel is available online at <http://www.nmc-uk.org/Employers-and-managers/Fitness-to-practise/> and further information on the outcomes of hearings of cases of alleged misconduct can be found at <http://www.nmc-uk.org/Hearings/Hearings-and-outcomes/>

In **Case study 5.2**, use of the Internet had a direct role to play.

Case study 5.2 Decision making and inappropriate behaviour

On 6 September 2010, Timothy Hyde, a community psychiatric nurse, was struck off for conducting an inappropriate relationship with a former patient. He had met Patient A when she attended a screening assessment, and he agreed to offer her counselling and

(Continued)

Case study 5.2 (Continued)

support. In the course of the therapeutic support, he learned that she had a history of difficult relationships and self-harm.

Two weeks after Patient A was discharged from the clinic, Hyde contacted her through Facebook. Over the following five weeks, they saw each other regularly and developed a sexual relationship, which Patient A eventually ended. She reported that Hyde had stated to her that he 'did not have space for someone like her in his life' and that he took the step of blocking her on Facebook. She later told her treating psychologist that she considered that Hyde had used his knowledge of her when choosing his parting words to her and that such comments had led her to a further episode of self-harm.

In reaching a decision that Hyde's behaviour amounted to misconduct, the Fitness to Practise panel stated that:

> As the code makes clear, nurses are required to be responsible for their actions, act with integrity and uphold the good standing of the profession.
>
> A nurse must at all times maintain appropriate professional boundaries in the relationship they have with patients and clients. He must ensure that all aspects of the relationship focus exclusively on the patient or client.
>
> Further, nurses must not abuse their privileged position for their own ends.

In deciding to 'strike him off'—that is, to remove his name from the register of nurses—the panel concluded that:

> ... the registrant's conduct displays a fundamental incompatibility with continued inclusion on the nursing register. The panel is of the view that the registrant's conduct was exploitative of a vulnerable client who had very recently been under his care. His wholly inappropriate engagement in an emotional and sexual relationship with patient A caused actual harm to her.
>
> (Jaeger 2011: 3–4)

Issue to Consider

Reflecting on this case study, ask yourself the following question: what aspects of human behaviour irritate you or give you cause for concern?

Your answer to the question in **Case study 5.2** may have included ignorance, rudeness, disrespect, discrimination, verbal, physical or mental abuse, violence, cheating, bullying, theft, laziness, fraud, or dishonesty.

In caring for members of the public, you meet all kinds of people displaying a variety of behaviours. However, one common strand that probably draws them together is that they, the public, will expect the highest standards of conduct from you as you care for them. You will be expected to treat people as individuals and to respect their dignity, being polite, kind, caring, and compassionate at all times, even when you do not feel like it. In deciding to become a nurse, you have accepted that this demanding guidance applies to you.

The second part of this chapter brings together all of the issues discussed in the first part, by exploring a range of case studies that illustrate various decision-making situations involving professional values and related competencies. They focus on academic and practice issues.

The case studies

These various case studies, set in both university and clinical contexts, are intended to help you to discover your role as a student nurse and what decisions are appropriate in a variety of different situations with which you might be faced. The scenarios are based on real-life situations, but all of the names are fictitious.

Please note, however, that examples of real practitioners' cases that can be found on the NMC's website do refer to the practitioners by name. It is a matter of public protection that such information is readily available both to members of the public and the profession. There is no anonymity if registrants are found to have impaired fitness to practise as a result of misconduct or incompetence.

The scenarios here will be accompanied by examples of potential responses to decisions, with accompanying rationale or evidence. This will offer you, as a student, potential feedback on your actions or what actually happened with outcomes, so that you can appreciate whether the decision you made was an effective or ineffective one.

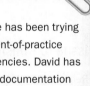

Case study 5.3 Falsifying a mentor's signature

David is a third-year pre-registration student on his final placement. He has been trying to find time to sit down with his mentor to complete David's assessment-of-practice documentation. His mentor has already signed off some of the proficiencies. David has already made an appointment to see his personal tutor to sign off his documentation at the university. This appointment is a week before the submission date, because his personal tutor is going on annual leave before that date.

The day on which David planned to meet with his mentor arrives, but his mentor has telephoned in sick. David is disappointed, because, based on what his mentor had been saying to him, he was confident that his documentation would be completed without any problems. The ward manager is unable to say when his mentor will be returning to the ward. David decides to sign off the outstanding proficiencies himself. He meets with his personal tutor, who is suspicious about some of the signatures on the document. His personal tutor telephones the placement to speak to David's mentor, but discovers that the mentor has been off sick since before the date of sign-off recorded in David's assessment-of-practice documentation.

(Continued)

Case study 5.3 (Continued)

Questions

1. Why do you think David has decided to sign his own assessment-of-practice documents?
2. What do you think is going to happen now? Refer to your own university policies regarding such behaviour and the possible outcomes.
3. What would you decide to do? What do you think David should do now?
4. Is there anything that David should and could have done differently?
5. Is this behaviour misconduct?
6. If you think it is, why have you come to that conclusion?
7. Review the NMC's Guidance (NMC 2011) to determine which areas of good health, good character, and fitness to practise David has breached through this behaviour and the decision to sign off his own proficiencies.

Issues to consider

It is clear from the NMC's Guidance (NMC 2011: 7) that David's decision is, in fact, an instance of cheating or plagiarism and that it is an area of cause for concern that would have had serious consequences for David. He is also fraudulently signing someone else's name.

Case study 5.4 Poor team work in classroom activity

Suzie is a second-year pre-registration student who is struggling with the academic workload of the programme. She is not able to manage her time effectively and is failing to produce the necessary feedback for her colleagues in her group. One of the members of the group, Lars, used to be her close friend, but ceased to be so after a disagreement about a mutual friend.

Lars is pretty fed up that Suzie has repeatedly let the group down by her failure to engage with the topic areas that she has been given.

Lars has shared his frustration with other group members and discovers that this is not the first time that some students in the group have been let down by Suzie. Lars plans to speak to the module leader about Suzie's failure to turn up for problem-based learning group sessions and her failure to do her share of the work.

(Continued)

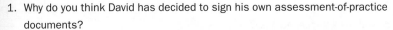

Case study 5.4 (Continued)

Questions

1. What would you do if you were Suzie?
2. What do you think happened next?
3. What would you decide to do if you were the module leader?
4. Is this behaviour misconduct?
5. If you think it is, why have you come to that conclusion?
6. Which components of the NMC (2011) *Guidance on Professional Conduct for Nursing and Midwifery Students* has Suzie breached through this behaviour?

Issues to consider

If you had responsibility for leading the group's activity, how would you feel about Suzie's decision not to produce the necessary feedback for her peers? It is important to remember that being a student nurse means getting involved and learning to contribute to a team approach: working together in the classroom helps you to learn team work decision-making skills.

Because Suzie has not completed work agreed with the group on a number of occasions, this behaviour could constitute what the NMC (2011: 8) calls 'persistent inappropriate attitude or behaviour'. It is evident that Suzie needs to make a decision, as well ask for help from her tutors, because she is apparently struggling with her academic work generally and with managing her time. There are many resources that universities have in place to help her in both of these areas of her student life.

Case study 5.5 Persistent use of a mobile phone in the classroom

Anna has been told on several occasions by university lecturers not to use her mobile phone while attending theoretical sessions in the classroom and lecture theatre. This behaviour continues to recur until a session facilitated by an outside speaker, who asked Anna to stop using her phone.

Anna responded by saying that she needed to keep her phone on because of issues in her home life. She continued using her mobile phone, disrupting the concentration of her peers. The speaker again asked Anna to stop using her phone and, when she refused, the speaker confiscated the phone.

(Continued)

Case study 5.5 (Continued)

Questions

1. What would you have done if you were Anna?
2. What do you think will happen now?
3. What would you do now if you were Anna?
4. Is this behaviour misconduct?
5. If you think it is, why have you come to that conclusion?
6. Which components of the NMC (2011) *Guidance on Professional Conduct for Nursing and Midwifery Students* has Anna breached through this behaviour?

Issues to consider

Here, again, we have a situation of persistent inappropriate attitude and behaviour by Anna, which is in effect disrupting the learning of the other students (NMC 2011: 8). Lecturers have discussed the issue of her using a mobile phone inappropriately in class on many occasions. Confiscating her mobile phone means, of course, that the outside speaker now has to take further action, and it could also be that Anna is angry and upset by the action. However, if this behaviour has been persistent, then again it is evident that Anna should expect there to be some consequences for her behaviour—possibly in the form of disciplinary action, and/or interviews with her personal teacher and programme leader.

It is not possible, of course, for us to see here all of the issues surrounding this scenario or any of the others, but it gives us an opportunity to consider different options for decisions made by students and others in the case study description.

Case study 5.6 A possible case of bullying and aggressive behaviour

Marsha is a second-year student, who is currently on a clinical placement with one of her peers, Barbara. They have not enjoyed an easy relationship when at the university: Marsha has regularly taunted Barbara about her weight and has made derogatory remarks about her appearance. Barbara appreciates that she should have taken a more assertive stand with Marsha prior to going to the clinical placement and regrets that she did not speak to university staff about how Marsha has treated her. Whilst on the placement, Barbara claims to have witnessed Marsha handling a child roughly and shouting at children in the playroom. Barbara decides to talk to her mentor about Marsha's behaviour.

(Continued)

Case study 5.6 (Continued)
Questions

1. What would you do if you were Marsha? What could have led to her decision to act as she has towards Barbara?
2. What do you think will happen now?
3. What would you decide to do if you were Barbara?
4. Is Marsha's behaviour a case of misconduct?
5. If you think it is, why have you come to that conclusion?
6. Which components of the NMC (2011) *Guidance on Professional Conduct for Nursing and Midwifery Students* has Marsha breached through this behaviour?

Issues to consider

Because there are two students involved in this scenario, we can also consider the decisions made here by Barbara. Although we have only some of the context information in this case study, we can see that it appears that Marsha could be bullying Barbara, because of the taunts about her weight and her appearance. She therefore has what could be reasons for 'getting back' at Marsha for her previous behaviour towards her, by making a serious practice allegation against Marsha in relation to her management of children in her care in the clinical placement. She makes the decision, however, to speak to her mentor about what she claims she has seen.

It could also be that as Barbara regrets not talking to someone in the university about Marsha's bullying behaviour and that her apparent experience of seeing Marsha exhibit a lack of care and potential 'aggressive, violent or threatening behaviour' (NMC 2011: 8) towards a child makes her realize that, this time, she has to speak to someone, given the potential seriousness of Marsha's behaviour and her practice as a student nurse.

Case study 5.7 Health matters and poor application to work

Katie is a second-year student who began the programme with great enthusiasm eighteen months ago. She enjoys the social life of a university student to the full, often burning the candle at both ends. Katie passed all of her assessments in the first year without any problems, although she readily admits that her success was good fortune rather than the result of consistent study.

Her progress in the second year has not been quite so easy. She is currently facing two theoretical resubmissions and her mentor has contacted her personal tutor to express concern about Katie's performance in practice. She has attended her placement sporadically and, when she does attend, she is invariably late. She is paying

(Continued)

Case study 5.7 (Continued)

minimal attention to her personal hygiene and frequently appears to be sleepy. She has also been short-tempered with her colleagues and has failed to follow instructions in relation to client care.

Questions

1. What would you have done if you were Katie?
2. What do you think will happen now?
3. What would you decide to do now if you were Katie?
4. Is Katie's behaviour misconduct?
5. If you think it is, why have you come to that conclusion?
6. Which components of the NMC (2011) *Guidance on Professional Conduct for Nursing and Midwifery Students* has Katie breached through this behaviour?

Issues to consider

It is apparent that Katie has managed to place herself in what may seem to be a cycle of inappropriate decisions, resulting in another cycle of behaviour affecting her whole life, not only her academic work. Her social life appears to be having a major impact on both her academic work and now her practice learning, and her increasing disinterest in both her practice as a student nurse and her personal health and well-being. The NMC (2011: 8) is clear that health concerns that have an impact on others, especially 'when there is a risk of harm to others', are an issue for 'fitness to practise' decisions, as is 'lack of insight into health concerns where there is a risk of harm to others'. Katie is also exhibiting 'poor application to work'.

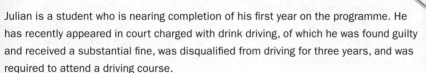

Case study 5.8 Non-declaration of a police conviction

Julian is a student who is nearing completion of his first year on the programme. He has recently appeared in court charged with drink driving, of which he was found guilty and received a substantial fine, was disqualified from driving for three years, and was required to attend a driving course.

He has recently failed to attend sessions at the university and has not contacted the programme support staff to explain his absence. All students in his cohort have recently been asked to submit their annual self-declaration in relation to cautions and convictions. Julian signs the form declaring no cautions or convictions. Two weeks later, his partner contacts the head of school to advise him of Julian's drink-driving conviction.

(Continued)

Case study 5.8 (Continued)

Questions

1. What would you have done if you were Julian?
2. What do you think will happen now?
3. What would you decide to do now if you were Julian?
4. Is this behaviour misconduct?
5. If you think it is, why have you come to that conclusion?
6. Which components of the NMC (2011) *Guidance on Professional Conduct for Nursing and Midwifery Students* has Julian breached through this behaviour?

Issues to consider

It is not an easy question in any of these case studies to imagine that you are the person who is the focus of the 'fitness for practice' concerns and you might even have thought, in reading the others, that 'It isn't going to happen to me' or 'I wouldn't put myself in that situation'.

However, it is clear from the information that we have that Julian has made some very serious decisions, the consequences of which he must now address personally and, of course, professionally in his learning journey to becoming a nurse. The situation described in relation to his drink-driving conviction is clearly a case of misconduct, which will result in a severe penalty for Julian—that is, dismissal from the programme. His poor attendance at the university, as well as fraudulent behaviour in non-declaration, simply adds to the 'fitness to practise' evidence.

Case study 5.9 Failure to declare a criminal conviction

Mandy is a mature student who has opted for a career in nursing after holding various jobs in the retail sector while bringing up her children. She made a decision not to fully disclose the circumstances of her past at the time of application. She failed to disclose a criminal conviction for shoplifting that she received when she was 17 years old. She has just attended a lecture entitled 'Professionalism', during which the lecturer reminded the audience that, for nurses, no criminal convictions are ever spent under the Rehabilitation of Offenders Act 1974.

Questions

1. What would you have done if you were Mandy?
2. What do you think will happen now?
3. What would you decide to do now if you were Mandy?
4. Is this behaviour misconduct?

(Continued)

Case study 5.9 (Continued)

5. If you think it is, why have you come to that conclusion?
6. Which components of the NMC (2011) *Guidance on Professional Conduct for Nursing and Midwifery Students* has Mandy breached through this behaviour?

Issues to consider

As with Julian's example, Mandy has failed to declare a previous criminal conviction for shoplifting received when she was younger (17 years old). In her case, the problem is not only that she had a conviction, but also that she knew that she should have declared it in her application form to become a nurse. She is now in a lecture in which she learns that not only is she in breach of university policy and the NMC (2011) professional conduct requirements, but also that her decision to not declare her previous conviction could be viewed as a 'fraudulent application form', and could put into question her 'fitness to practise' as a student and qualified nurse.

In all of these case studies, many issues have been raised that require much more thought and also more information than is possible to include in this chapter. It is hoped that, by reading them, you will have been able to see how decisions by all of the individuals concerned not only affect each of them, but also others. Use them to discuss with your mentors and colleagues the importance of the *Guidance on Professional Conduct for Nursing and Midwifery Students* (NMC 2011).

It is important that you are aware that your behaviour and conduct, both during your programme and in your personal life, may have an impact on your fitness to practise. Students should be reminded that it is their responsibility to inform the university if they receive a charge, conviction, or caution during their programme, or if they develop a health condition or disability that may affect their ability to practise safely and effectively.

....

Top Tips

What can student nurses do to ensure that they develop appropriate professional conduct?

1. Work through the case studies in this chapter.
2. Ensure that you are familiar with the guidance that is published by the NMC both for student nurses and midwives, and for registered practitioners.
3. Ensure that you are familiar with the policies and procedures of your university and your clinical placements.
4. Reflect upon your own professional conduct and behaviour.
5. Seek support from your university via your personal tutors, academic supervisors, programme leaders, and your peers about professional conduct matters that concern you.
6. Participate in discussions regarding professional behaviour and conduct.

7. When on placement, seek support from your mentor/assessor and other practice-based staff who have been identified as sources of support for students if you are concerned about issues that have arisen with clients.
8. At any time that you are in doubt about any aspect of your practice, raise your concerns with an appropriate member of staff.
9. Remember that staff at your university and in your practice placements are keen to help you to achieve your aspiration to become a registered nurse.

Conclusion

This chapter has focused on the first of the NMC Standards (2010)—namely, the domain entitled 'Professional values'. It has not been possible to cover every aspect of the NMC (2011) Guidance, nor all of the competencies that you have to achieve to become a registered nurse. It is important to remember that any decision that you make that impacts on your development of professional practice to become a nurse also includes maintaining a high standard of practice and care to your patients and clients at all times.

References

Jaeger, A. (2011) 'Facebook trials and tribulations: social networking sites and their joys and dangers', NMC Factsheet, available online at <http://www.nmc-uk.org/Documents/Events/Staff-at-events/Handout_Facebook-trials-and-tribulations-social-networking-sites-and-their-joys-and-dangers.PDF>

Nursing and Midwifery Council (2008) *The Code: Standards of Conduct, Performance and Ethics for Nurses and Midwives*, London: NMC.

Nursing and Midwifery Council (2010) *Standards for Pre-Registration Nursing Education*, London: NMC.

Nursing and Midwifery Council (2011) *Guidance on Professional Conduct for Nursing and Midwifery Students*, London: NMC.

Further Reading

Sellman, D. (2007) 'On being of good character: nurse education and the assessment of good character', *Nurse Education Today*, 27(7): 762–7.

Useful Links and Resources

<http://www.nmc-uk.org/Documents/Guidance/NMC-Guidance-on-professional-conduct-for-nursing-and-midwifery-students.PDF>

The NMC's *Guidance on Professional Conduct for Nursing and Midwifery Students* (2011).

<http://www.nmc-uk.org/Hearings/>

The NMC publishes details of all proceedings heard at professional misconduct hearings.

<http://www.nmc-uk.org/Students/Top-resources-for-students/>

This useful page of the NMC site provides guidance and resources for student nurses.

6

Communication, interpersonal skills, and decision making

Jenni Templeman and June Keeling

The aims of this chapter are to:

➔ explore a range of communication strategies as they relate to decision making;

➔ explore how communication skills can influence how we relate to others through our interpersonal skills;

➔ use case studies to explore how student nurses can meet the Nursing and Midwifery Council competencies in 'Communication and interpersonal skills'; and

➔ explore how effective communication and interpersonal skills are essential in decision-making situations in nursing practice.

Introduction

This chapter explores the various aspects of communication and how these relate to our own interpersonal skills in communicating with others. The effectiveness of our communication—that is, how good we are at passing on information and ensuring that another person understands what we are trying to say—has a direct effect on both our own decision-making skills and the decisions made by those around us.

We have all come across health care professionals whom we have felt have a good 'bedside manner' and those who do not. Historically, this term has been used to describe those who can communicate effectively. It is very important that, through our use of words, the person listening is able to understand what we mean. In nursing and health care generally, there is an increasing emphasis on communication as a means of building therapeutic relationships with both patients and their relatives.

Communication, in the light of new technologies and ease of access by the wider community, extends far beyond the patient's reliance on others for information about his or her health and well-being. It now encompasses more interpersonal communication, in which patients can be viewed as 'the expert' in conversations with nurses and doctors, an increased awareness of cultural influences, and the use of social networking sites, as well as the numerous Internet sites now available, to offer possible diagnoses and treatment options for the general public.

Making decisions about patients' health and often whether to accept those made on their behalf by others is now a real challenge for health professionals when communicating with patients and their families. As a nurse, it is part of your role to make decisions *with* patients and their families not *for* them, and the importance of learning how to communicate effectively, as well as how to engage in communicating with people, is clearly evident in the fact that the Nursing and Midwifery Council (NMC) *Standards for Pre-Registration Nursing Education* (NMC 2010b) now includes a new set of competencies solely for 'Communication and interpersonal skills'.

The Nursing and Midwifery Council Standards (2010) and Essential Skills Clusters

Currently in nursing practice, the student nurse needs to acquire the competence and skills to communicate effectively, as well as those related to decision making (NMC 2010b). The majority of complaints within the National Health Service (NHS) originate from ineffective communication between health care staff and the patient and relatives (Pincock 2004). Therefore we suggest that central to all decision making in practice settings is patient-centred communication—that is, communication that is centred around the patient and his or her relatives. Our honesty, trust, and respect for each individual patient's cultural values and beliefs, along with a genuine concern for his or her well-being, enables the patient to participate with confidence in the care that he or she is receiving.

The NMC stipulates specific standards of competence that are deemed necessary for the delivery of safe, effective nursing practice. Additionally, it also identifies specific skills that nursing students must achieve throughout their training programme, known as 'essential skills clusters' (ESCs).

The NMC's *Standards for Pre-Registration Nursing Education* (NMC 2010b), 'Domain 2: Communication and interpersonal skills—Generic standard for competence', specifies that:

> *All nurses must use excellent communication and interpersonal skills. Their communications must always be safe, effective, compassionate and respectful. They must communicate effectively using a wide range of strategies and interventions, including effective use of communication technologies. Where people have a disability, nurses must be able to work with service users and others to obtain the information needed to make reasonable adjustments that promote optimum health and enable equal access to services.*
>
> (NMC 2010b: 15)

The ESC entitled 'Care, compassion and communication' recommends that, in relation to communication skills, the newly qualified nurse should provide care that is therapeutic, and underpinned by effective listening and oral skills, as well as provide information 'that is clear and free from jargon'. (See **Box 6.1** and **Table 6.1** for the exact skills that you will be expected to have attained at the three assessment points in your curriculum in order to enter into the register as a nurse.) The way in which you can learn to achieve these skills, and the generic and field-specific competencies related to communication and decision making, will be explored throughout this chapter.

To achieve this learning, we will explore the many different facets of communication, interpersonal skills, and decision making, using clinical case studies to encourage the reader to *stop* and *think*, together with different activities related to the case studies. Each of these aspects has been explored as a separate theme to assist in the clarity of the reading, but it is important to acknowledge that they are all interlinked in health care.

The chapter includes case studies that explore the fundamental aspects of effective communication, interpersonal skills, and decision making within clinical practice in terms of:

- communicating with colleagues (including communication in difficult circumstances, challenging others, and interpersonal decision making);
- communicating with patients and carers (learning through observation);
- therapeutic relationships and professional boundaries (making the right decisions);
- communicating through various technologies and decision making (social networking sites and issues of confidentiality linked to professional values);
- the importance of effective communication in the delivery of quality health care to patients and their relatives/significant others; and
- examples from student nurses and newly qualified nurses to illustrate the nature of decisions that may be required in relation to the competencies at different stages of your programme.

In order to ensure that you have a common understanding of what we mean by 'communication' and 'interpersonal skills' in the context of decision making and therapeutic practice as a nurse, we will initially explore these as they have been defined in the literature.

Box 6.1 Essential skills cluster: Care compassion and communication

6 *People can trust the newly registered graduate nurse to engage therapeutically and actively listen to their needs and concerns, responding using skills that are helpful, providing information that is clear, accurate, meaningful and free from jargon.*

Table 6.1 Essential skills clusters at progression points 1, 2, and 3

First progression point	Second progression point	Entry to the register
1 Communicates effectively both orally and in writing, so that the meaning is always clear.	6 Uses strategies to enhance communication and remove barriers to effective communication minimising risk to people from lack of or poor communication.	7 Consistently shows ability to communicate safely and effectively with people providing guidance for others.
2 Records information accurately and clearly on the basis of observation and communication.		8 Communicates effectively and sensitively in different settings, using a range of methods and skills.
3 Always seeks to confirm understanding.		9 Provides accurate and comprehensive written and verbal reports based on best available evidence.
4 Responds in a way that confirms what a person is communicating.		10 Acts autonomously to reduce and challenge barriers to effective communication and understanding.
5 Effectively communicates people's stated needs and wishes to other professionals.		11 Is proactive and creative in enhancing communication and understanding.
		12 Uses the skills of active listening, questioning, paraphrasing and reflection to support a therapeutic intervention.

Source: NMC (2010b: Annexe 3)

Communication and interpersonal skills

As noted, communication and interpersonal skills competencies are the focus of Domain 2 of the NMC Standards (NMC 2010b). Both of these are fundamental to our achieving the other three domains—that is, 'Professional values', 'Nursing practice and decision making', and 'Leadership, management and team working'—because most of the competencies in these three areas involve some kind of communication.

In our development as human beings, one of the first skills that we learned was to communicate ideas through the medium of language, which we developed and refined from mere sounds to form commonly understood words and phrases (Bach and Grant 2010). Over time, our methods of communication for language in the written and spoken form have become sophisticated, especially in the present day when we have highly technological methods at our disposal, such as electronic formatted communication, the Internet, the workplace intranet, and social networking sites (Webb 2011). There are so many different facets of communication involved in clinical practice that it would be impossible to define them all, but we can consider more general definitions.

Balzer-Riley (2004: 6) considers that 'Communication involves the reciprocal process in which messages are sent and received between two or more people', while Hargie and Dickson (2004: 41) in turn suggest that 'interpersonal communication can be thought of as a process that is transactional, purposeful, multi-dimensional, irreversible and (possibly) inevitable'.

Activity

Webb (2011) offers further examples of different models of communication, discusses theories of interpersonal skills, and explores briefly their use in nursing practice. Access the Online Resource Centre that accompanies the book (see the end of the chapter for the web link) and read the sample chapter.

This site also offers you the opportunity to access a range of additional resources to support your learning about communication and interpersonal skills in a wide range of nursing and health care situations. These will also be of value in other sections of this chapter, as well as throughout this book itself.

Nursing involves the need for good communication skills that have a therapeutic effect on the delivery of good care, because nurses who can communicate at an emotional level are seen as warm, caring, and empathetic (Webb 2011). Nurses who possess these qualities of warmth, caring, and empathy instil trust and confidence in their patients, which can enable the patient to disclose any concerns, to ask questions about his or her condition, to become involved in the available treatment options, and to develop a greater understanding of them in order to self-care.

Research suggests that when nurses provide a good environment, use therapeutic communication, and give accurate information, patients experience positive health benefits such as reduced pain and lowered blood pressure (Kwekkeboom 1997; Webb 2011). The patient profile in current nursing practice is a complex blend of both acute and chronic illness, with an emphasis on patient choice, self-care, individual patient preference, and the patient's values and expectations with regard to treatment options.

Both written and spoken communication is an important way of transmitting vital information about patient issues in nursing. It is through effective and good communication, and the development of the therapeutic relationship between a nurse and a patient, that nurses can identify the unique individual needs of a patient (Foy and Timmins 2004; Sharples and Elcock 2011). Patients need to be listened to, need to feel that their concerns are being addressed, need to be supported, and need to feel understood within this therapeutic relationship (Gilbert and Leahy 2007). Some nurses are naturally gifted in communication skills, while others have to learn and master the skill.

Verbal communication

As human beings, we use verbal communication in every aspect of our daily lives, so it is surprising that we are not experts in this particular skill.

Communication lies at the heart of nursing and, together with interpersonal skills and decision-making skills, underpins all phases of clinical practice for both student nurses and qualified nurses. Communication and interpersonal skills are inseparable from the care and compassion that we give to our patients. Effective communication is a continuous thread and theme throughout nursing, and, together with interpersonal skills, fosters quality and competent caring (Sharples and Elcock 2011). Communication (both verbal and written) is a prerequisite to competent nursing practice, because it is a way of transmitting vital information about our patients in our care and documenting the findings.

As a nurse, you use verbal communication on a daily basis, but often this information is misunderstood. Miscommunication of patient information occurs, which may lead to health errors and can be detrimental to patient care. These mistakes are sometimes evident in the adherence to times for medication administration. Within the health care setting, students need to adjust to different clinical placement environments, each with their own particular jargon and specialist language. In the specialized area of theatre, voices are often muffled as a result of the face masks worn in this area. The nursing and medical personnel also speak in their 'theatre' jargon, which may be misinterpreted and not understood. This specialized jargon and language is apparent in each of the speciality disciplines within health care practice. This concept of new or unfamiliar language and terminology within health care is often different from the language that students use in their off-duty time. During your professional development, you may experience a lack of communication confidence, which may lead to a certain degree of stress, anxiety, and lack of confidence. However, the best way of improving your verbal communication skills is to develop your listening skills (Sharples and Elcock 2011).

Active listening

In order to develop your listening skills, you will need to develop your *active* listening skills, because the reason that you speak is to pass on information to other people. Miscommunication will occur if the information that you pass on is not clear or clearly understood. Hearing is part of active listening, as is the recognition of non-verbal communication, often referred to as 'body language' (McCabe and Timmins 2006). Always check that information has been clearly delivered in your communication with both patients and colleagues.

Active listening means that you are paying attention to what is being said and also to how it is being said (Sharples and Elcock 2011). Eye contact, head-nodding, and facial expressions are body postures and gestures that may give you an indication of whether your communication is clear and you are being understood. In clinical practice, a nurse may ask the patient if he or she has understood what has been explained, because active listening is a deliberate commitment to engage fully with everyone—colleagues, patients, and staff (Foy and Timmins 2004). Active listening also involves being able to remain silent and allow the other person to speak. Nurses sometimes have difficulty in maintaining silence, especially when breaking bad news (see **Box 6.2**).

Box 6.2 Active listening

Active listening involves:
- *looking directly at the person when you are speaking and when he or she is speaking to you;*
- *not interrupting people when they are speaking;*
- *observing their body language and taking note of what they are saying;*
- *reflecting your feelings in your body language and facial expression; and*
- *observing people for feedback with regard to your communication.*

(McCabe and Timmins 2006)

Having considered the main types of communication skill required as a nurse and how you might approach the interpersonal aspects of communication, we can explore some possible scenarios that you may come across in practice placements and elsewhere in your learning experience.

To ensure that your professional accountability, and personal knowledge and development are considered, please access (using the links that you will find at the end of the chapter) and read the NMC's *Record Keeping Guidance for Nurses and Midwives* (NMC 2010a) and the *Standards for Pre-Registration Nursing Education* (NMC 2010b), including the competencies for 'Communication and interpersonal skills' and the ESCs for 'Care, compassion and communication'. Use these to help you to consider how the case studies can help you to meet your communication competencies.

We have also included further reading for you in relation to all of the case studies. Consider **Case study 6.1**.

Case study 6.1 Communicating with a dying person

An 80-year-old man recently diagnosed with terminal cancer is admitted to the oncology ward for pain management. Jo, a third-year student nurse, is conducting his admission in a friendly, yet professional, manner. The patient says to Jo: 'I want to die at home in my own surroundings, not in hospital. I know I'm going to die soon . . .'.

Jo is a little taken aback by this statement, but remembers what she has been taught about active listening skills and showing warmth, empathy, and friendliness towards patients who put their trust in a nurse. So Jo draws the curtains around the patient's bed to maintain privacy and moves the chair closer to the patient. She holds his hand

(Continued)

Case Study 6.1 (Continued)

and asks him if he would like to talk about his feelings related to his statement. Jo maintains eye contact with the patient, and makes sure that her facial expressions and gestures reflect her interest in and understanding of what the patient is saying. Jo's professional and friendly manner has developed into a trusting and respectful therapeutic relationship between herself and the patient. The patient asks Jo a few questions that she cannot answer, so she suggests that the patient ask her mentor, who is a qualified palliative care nurse, and the doctor.

After their discussion, Jo tells the patient that she has documented his request in his case notes and that, with his permission, she will discuss his request with her mentor. Jo and her mentor then arrange a meeting between the doctor and the patient to enable him to discuss his concerns and his request to die at home. The patient gives his permission for Jo to discuss his request and concerns with her mentor.

Questions

Identify the main issues in this case study and consider the following questions.

1. Do you think that Jo's active listening skills were effective?
2. Did Jo adhere to the NMC's *Guidance on Professional Conduct for Nursing and Midwifery Students* (NMC 2009) with regard to confidentiality and disclosure?
3. In what other ways could Jo support the patient with regard to seeking more information?
4. Do you think that holding a patient's hand could be therapeutic?
5. Would you feel comfortable talking to a patient about dying and death?

Written communication

During your course of study, there are numerous opportunities for you learn about written communication and how to document aspects of patient care, and your own personal and professional development. The student nurse learns how to document patient's notes, records, charts, and nursing care plans under the supervision and guidance of a mentor or registered nurse. There are legal and ethical reasons why student nurses are guided by their mentors and/or other registered nurses when completing documentation with regards to patient care. The student nurse's documentation and record-keeping is always reviewed and countersigned by a qualified nurse. Once qualified, the nurse is professionally accountable and responsible for his or her acts and omissions regarding documentation and record-keeping according to the laws of the country and the NMC (NMC 2009).

As a student nurse, you will have had numerous opportunities to practise your verbal skills independently, but will not have had the same opportunities for independent practice with record-keeping. (See Webb 2011 and its accompanying Online Resource Centre for further information on record-keeping. You will find the link at the end of the chapter.)

Once you are qualified as a registered nurse, your literacy will be judged in terms of your ability to deliver high-quality care, as evidenced by concrete skills such as your charting ability, record-keeping and writing ability, and patient assessment (Anders et al. 1995; Learner 2006; Sharples and Elcock 2011). To explore this issue of documentation as communication, consider **Case study 6.2**.

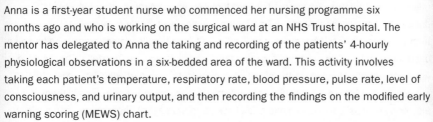

Case study 6.2 Documenting patient observations

Anna is a first-year student nurse who commenced her nursing programme six months ago and who is working on the surgical ward at an NHS Trust hospital. The mentor has delegated to Anna the taking and recording of the patients' 4-hourly physiological observations in a six-bedded area of the ward. This activity involves taking each patient's temperature, respiratory rate, blood pressure, pulse rate, level of consciousness, and urinary output, and then recording the findings on the modified early warning scoring (MEWS) chart.

Mr Robin is an older person in bed 5 who underwent abdominal surgery two days ago, and who has an intravenous infusion and urinary catheter in situ, a nasogastric tube on free drainage, and a large abdominal wound. Anna introduces herself to the patient and requests permission to conduct the observations. She makes sure that the patient is comfortable before proceeding. Prior to and after taking his observations, Anna checks the patient's name, age, and patient number on both the chart and the patient's armband. Whilst documenting the observations on the MEWS chart, Anna notices that the patient's MEWS score is triggering 7, and his pulse and respiratory rate have increased with a low blood pressure. The patient's urine in the catheter bag is also rather dark and concentrated. Anna remembers that a score of 3 is normal for the MEWS assessment, because this was taught at the university and also by her mentor on the ward. Anna makes the patient comfortable after taking his observations and hurries off to report the MEWS chart findings to her mentor.

Questions

Identify the main issues in this case study and consider the following questions.
1. Do you think that Anna responded correctly by reporting the patient's findings immediately?

(Continued)

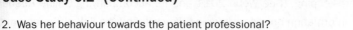

Case Study 6.2 (Continued)

2. Was her behaviour towards the patient professional?
3. Did she act within her scope of practice as a student nurse according to *The Code: Standards of Conduct, Performance and Ethics for Nurses and Midwives* (NMC 2008)?
4. The mentor immediately reviewed the patient and contacted the outreach team, because the patient's condition could deteriorate rapidly and put him in danger. The outreach nurse assessed the patient, and prescribed additional intravenous fluids for the patient and hourly observations. Why do you think the outreach nurse prescribed additional fluids and hourly observations?

Issues to consider

Anna's mentor thanked her for responding so swiftly and for acting in an intelligent and efficient way. This was documented in Anna's placement document, where she was duly praised for her diligence. At the university, the practice lead and Anna's personal academic tutor also congratulated her on her excellent report from the placement area. Anna has also used this event as one of her written reflections on practice for her portfolio. This enabled Anna and her tutor to discuss the situation in more detail—in particular, how what she has recorded not only showed how she had undertaken observations and recorded them, but also how she was learning to make a link between physiological observations and decision making, resulting in prompt action to ensure the safety of the patient in her care.

Do you think communication between the practice placement area and the university has a positive impact on the student nurse's progress? Think of a time when you were praised for acting responsibly and intelligently. How did you feel?

Using one of the reflective frameworks in **Chapter 4**, reflect on a recent written example of your documentation and compare it with past examples of written documentation (for example, compare your documentation from the first year to that produced during your second and/or third years). Has your documentation and writing ability changed and improved?

We can see from the example in **Case study 6.2** that communication of different kinds are inextricably linked with decision making, but as Anna showed by immediately reporting her findings to her mentor, she made the decision within her own limits of competence and therefore the NMC Guidance (NMC 2009).

Communicating through social networking sites

The rapid development and use of social networking sites, and the facility of instant messaging, has expanded exponentially in recent years. Recent estimates of this usage include 500 million users globally (Facebook 2011). Within the United Kingdom, 7,580 users identified their profession as a nurse, midwife, or health visitor (Facebook 2011), demonstrating the widespread use of this medium of communication. In fact, the NMC itself has its own Facebook page (**<http://www.facebook.com/ nmcuk>**). Social networking has been discussed in **Chapter 5**, in the context of the student nurse and maintaining professional values and behaviour; in this chapter, we recognize the importance of this growing area of uncertainty for many student nurses, and approach the issues from a communication and decision-making perspective. In this way, we hope to reaffirm the expectations that professional bodies worldwide, such as the NMC, have of all nurses in relation to professional behaviour and social media.

With the development of instant messaging, social networking sites, and other forms of online communication, we can transmit and receive information almost instantaneously. The information that we divulge may also be visible on personal websites and blogs, discussion boards, and emails. This also covers all kinds of content shared online, including text, photographs, images, video, and audio files. Increasingly, organizations rely on instant messaging to transmit information to large groups of people. The NMC and most universities also engage with the students in this way, as do many other professional bodies worldwide. At a more intrinsic level, we, as health care professionals, also use these media to communicate with our peers, family, and others, and therefore it is essential that we use them responsibly to ensure that our communications with others are within our professional code of conduct. This applies as much to students and qualified nurses and midwives working in other parts of the world as it does to those working in the UK.

Many students have, unfortunately, been disciplined on the basis of their fitness to practise as a student nurse because of issues arising as a consequence of an ill-thought-out comment, or the posting of an inappropriate photograph on a social networking site, or an inappropriate text to a 'friend'. The instantaneous nature of these networking sites leaves little time for us to reflect on our spontaneity when sending messages to others. (The key has been pressed before we have time to reconsider whether it is the right thing to do.)

The NMC (2012) clearly identifies that a health professional's behaviour in the 'real world' and that on social networking sites should be considered subject to the same professional acceptable standard, and that the same rules of conduct apply to both. The ever-increasing usage of social networking sites and the reliance on this form of rapid communication may result in this becoming an established method of communication between organizations and students, for example when their virtual online learning site is out of action and an urgent message is required to inform students of a change in their timetable. However, whilst the social norms of conduct and behaviour continue to evolve, the levels of acceptability in professional behaviours are a constant and should be adhered to at all times.

Box 6.3 lists some examples of the inappropriate use of social networking sites.

Box 6.3 Examples of inappropriate use of social networking sites

- *Posting inappropriate comments about colleagues or patients*
- *Use of social networking sites to bully or intimidate colleagues*
- *Pursuing personal relationships with patients or service users*
- *Distributing sexually explicit material*
- *Using social networking sites in any way that is unlawful*
- *Manipulated photos that are intended to mock individuals*

(NMC 2012)

It is essential to maintain effective professional communication at all times. We also need to be aware of the myths surrounding the acceptability of communication, particularly when using social networking sites, blogs, or instant messaging (see **Box 6.4**).

Box 6.4 Myths about social networking communications

- It is misguided to believe that any communication about work-related issues, including conversations about patients, complaints about colleagues, or the clinical area, are private and anonymous.
- It is misguided to believe that any communication via a social networking site, or through blogs, instant messaging, or Twitter, is private and accessible only to the intended recipient. Once the message has been posted, it can easily be disseminated to others.
- It is misguided to believe that sharing of patient information with another person is harmless even if that private information is disclosed to the intended recipient. This may still be a breach of confidentiality if the patient has not given his or her permission for this information to be shared.
- It is misguided to believe that you may communicate with patients and service users, even if they are no longer in your care.

Consider **Case study 6.3** in relation to confidentiality.

Case study 6.3 Confidentiality and professional practice

Tim, a registered learning disability nurse with ten years' experience working within the community, was leaving his post to take on new responsibilities. At a leaving party, he was co-supervising an outing to a ten-pin bowling alley. Tim used his mobile phone to take a picture of a service user and himself whilst on this outing. Prior to taking the photograph, Tim had asked the permission of the service user's mother, who had agreed to it being taken. A copy of the photograph was later given to both the service user and mother. A few weeks later, Tim's mobile phone, which contained the photo of the service user, was stolen. This photo was later seen on a social networking site.

Questions

Identify what you think are the main issues in this case study and consider the following observations in relation to the questions:

- there is a lack of confidentiality for the service user, because the photo is now in the public domain;
- the photograph should have been deleted as soon as it was used for the purpose for which consent had been given;
- there are issues of safeguarding if the service user or location is identifiable; and
- using a personal device to take a patient's photo is improper and not permitted.

1. Do nurses need to obtain valid consent before taking photographs of patients?
2. Should persons no longer involved in the care of the service user have access to personal and confidential information?

The NMC states that nurses should not take or keep photographs of any person, or his or her family, that are not clinically relevant (NMC 2009). You should take some time to reflect on this standard.

Communication and decision making

Communication and decision making are closely interwoven into daily nursing clinical practice. Decision making improves as the nurse gains more experience of nursing different patients, and incorporates intuition and evidence-based research as a source of knowledge and information.

According to Thompson and Dowding (2002), clinical decision making may be defined as choosing between alternatives. It is a process that, as nurses, we undertake on a daily basis when we make judgements about the care that we provide to our patients. It involves observation, critical thinking, evaluating the evidence, applying knowledge, problem-solving, reflection, and clinical judgement (Standing 2010). As nurses gain more experience, the process of clinical decision making becomes easier.

Decision making is a complex activity that also requires knowledge, intuition, and evidence-based practice based on robust research findings (see **Chapter 1**). The inexperienced or novice nurse is guided in clinical practice by the various protocols, guidelines, policies, and care pathways that can be used to make decisions, but as the nurse gains more experience, decision making becomes more intuitive. This is a process of both personal and professional development, which, with time, empowers our clinical practice and sharpens our decision-making skills. The student nurse is continually learning these skills through observing more experienced staff making decisions within clinical practice. Evidence-based practice is a process by which nurses and other health care practitioners make clinical decisions using the best available research evidence, their clinical expertise, and patient preferences (Thompson 2003).

Decision making as a process helps the nurse to select the best course of action that optimizes a patient's health and minimizes any harm (Standing 2010). The nurse is professionally accountable for accurately assessing a patient's needs using the appropriate sources of information and planning nursing interventions that address problems (Standing 2010). These decision-making competencies will be evaluated throughout the student nurse's programme, as their achievement of the competencies outlined in the NMC Standards (NMC 2010b) is assessed.

In current nursing practice, shared decision making with the service user is at the hub of patient-centred care and in keeping with nursing values (Sharples and Elcock 2011). The aim of the UK government's White Paper *Equity and Excellence: Liberating the NHS* (Department of Health 2010) is to empower patients to share in the decisions about their care. In current society, patients have a wealth of information at their disposal via the Internet, social networking sites, and mailing lists, and are much more informed about their health and well-being needs (O'Grady and Jadad 2010).

As a student nurse or newly qualified nurse, you may feel that you do not have the experience and knowledge to support patients in the decision-making process, but you should encourage them to become involved in their treatment and intervention options (Sharples and Elcock 2011). Additionally, nurses should include the patient in decision making around nursing interventions and lifestyle choices, as well as being an advocate in situations in which other health care professionals are not offering patients the opportunity for shared decision making (Sharples and Elcock 2011). Student nurses and newly qualified nurses are supported by mentors and preceptors in clinical situations that require decision making.

Consider **Case study 6.4**, which explores shared decision making.

Case study 6.4 Shared decision making

A 30-year-old man is being assessed in the accident and emergency (A&E) department by Michael, a newly qualified nurse. The patient has a high blood glucose level and is displaying signs of uncontrolled diabetes. In broken English, he informs Michael that he is an insulin-dependent diabetic from Poland and has been working in the United Kingdom for two months. After taking his history, it is clear that the patient has a problem speaking and understanding the English language. Michael contacts the hospital's Polish interpreter for further assistance in communicating with the patient. Michael realizes that, to help the patient to achieve a state of well-being and diabetic control, the patient will require acute medical intervention, diabetic education with regard to his medication, a referral to the hospital's diabetic dietician, and follow-up outpatient appointments. This will involve a collaborative team effort from Michael, the specialist diabetic nurse, the interpreter, the dietician, and the attending doctor in A&E. The team decides to admit the man for diabetic control and that further management will involve a multidisciplinary approach to support the patient on discharge.

Questions

Identify the main issues in this case study and consider the following questions.
1. Do you think a multidisciplinary approach will help the patient to achieve well-being?
2. Was Michael's decision effective in this scenario?
3. Reflect on the decision-making process adopted by Michael and consider a clinical decision that you have made recently. What was the decision about? What judgements led you to make this decision?
4. Access the Code (NMC 2008) and read what it has to say about advocacy, accountability, and responsibility.

Communication and therapeutic relationships

Communication is an essential component of nursing care that contributes to the attainment of an effective therapeutic relationship with a patient. McMahon (1998: 10) defines a 'therapeutic relationship' as one that can be seen to be 'achieving beneficial outcomes for the patient's problems, using interventions that acknowledge and complement the work of other therapists and with due regard for the goals and individuality of the patient'.

These goals may be learning to deal with a newly diagnosed life-limiting illness or beginning a long-term self-administration medication programme. Wosket (2006) argues that the efficacy of a therapeutic relationship may directly affect the outcomes. It is important to the success of the patient's journey that the nurse is able to demonstrate empathy, support, and information-giving, and to facilitate the development of a therapeutic relationship with the patient. Additionally, Owen (2004) identifies unconditional acceptance, attending and listening, open questioning, reflection, professionalism, and warmth and being genuine as key components to an effective relationship with a patient that becomes therapeutic. The ultimate aim of nurses using therapeutic communication skills is to provide a sense of well-being for patients by making them feel relaxed and secure (McCabe and Timmins 2006). This therapeutic relationship should encourage patient-centred communication in which the patient is respected as an individual and has control over the care that he or she receives.

Self-awareness is a critical feature in the development of therapeutic relationships. Nurses should be aware of their position or stance within the nurse–patient relationship and how they, as nurses, are perceived by others. Self-awareness is a significant tool for improving nurse–patient interaction and is integrated into nurse education programmes. Being self-aware as a nurse is essential for the successful implementation of the therapeutic relationship, and is important for a nurse's professional and personal development (McCabe and Timmins 2006).

Bach and Grant (2010) state that acknowledgement of our own values, attitudes, and beliefs as a nurse is necessary to ensure that we become sensitive to complex situations. Indeed, prejudice, language, stereotyping, and being judgemental are significant barriers to a therapeutic relationship and the subsequent associated decision making. Therapeutic communication results in a focused and purposeful relationship between a nurse and the patient that helps the nurse to assess, plan, implement, and evaluate the care needed by a patient in a safe and competent manner (McCabe and Timmins 2006). Roper et al. (2001) emphasized the need for patient participation and patient-centred care in nursing, in that their model allows for the specific assessment of an individual's needs and the importance of an interpersonal relationship between a patient and a nurse.

The NMC Standards (NMC 2010b) and competencies stress the importance of appropriate behaviour between nurses and patients, and stipulate that all nurses must use therapeutic principles to engage, maintain, and, where appropriate, disengage from professional caring relationships. They must also always respect professional boundaries.

Consider **Case study 6.5** with regards to this issue of respecting professional boundaries.

Case study 6.5 Maintaining professional boundaries

Josh is a second-year nurse who accompanies his mentor, a psychiatric community nurse, to assess a 36-year-old woman with a diagnosis of psychosis. The patient is compliant with her present medication, and is maintaining her autonomy and independence. She enjoys talking to Josh, because he reminds her of a previous partner, and she mentions that she feels relaxed and at ease discussing her problems and fears with him. On this particular day, Josh informs her that his placement is nearing completion in a few days. He reassures her that it has been a pleasure meeting her and that he wishes her well for the future. She is visibly upset that she will no longer see Josh and asks him if he would visit her on his days off. Josh agrees to do this without discussing this issue with his mentor.

Questions

Identify the main issues in this case study and consider the following questions.
1. Will Josh fail to maintain his professional boundary if he visits the patient at home?
2. Has Josh maintained professional practice and adherence to the NMC Code (NMC 2008)?
3. There are issues of personal safety that arise as a result of friends and family of the patient whom Josh may encounter. To what potential risks could Josh be exposed?
4. How should Josh have ended this therapeutic relationship?

Activity

Read Miller, E. and Nambiar-Greenwood, G. (2011) 'The nurse–patient relationship', in L. Webb (ed.) *Nursing: Communication Skills in Practice*, Oxford: Oxford University Press, pp. 20–32, to help you to determine the answer to these issues. In addition, revisit the NMC *Guidance on Professional Conduct* and read again the section on 'Maintaining clear professional boundaries' (NMC 2009: 12).

Conclusion

Throughout your learning experiences as a student nurse, you will learn to identify appropriate communication strategies in order to deliver safe and effective patient care, as well as those required to work together with your colleagues and other professionals in both practice and university environments. To develop your communication skills, you will need to self-assess and reflect on the effectiveness of your interpersonal skills. To achieve this, you will need to be knowledgeable with regard to the current NMC Standards and Guidance relevant to verbal and written communication and accurate record-keeping, as well as that impacting on relationships with others.

If ever you are in doubt with regard to making the right decision in any situation, then it is imperative that you seek guidance from more experienced colleagues, your personal tutor, or your mentor, depending, of course, on the kind of decision that is required. Decision making is an acquired skill, which is developed and refined through experience; as you gain more experience, so too will your confidence increase. You will be expected to achieve all of the generic and field-specific competencies relevant to the NMC Standards and the domain of 'Communication and interpersonal skills' (NMC 2010b). Developing your decision-making skills in communicating with people and through other means is essential for your successful attainment of these competencies. Reflecting on your communicating and interpersonal skills and experiences will facilitate the development of increasing confidence to manage complex decision-making situations, as required of the qualified nurse. This will benefit not only you, but ultimately the patients and clients in your care.

References

Anders, H., Douglas, D., and Harrigan, R. (1995) 'Competencies of new registered nurses: a survey of deans and health care agencies in the state of Hawaii', *Nursing Connections*, 8(3): 5–16.

Bach, S. and Grant, A. (2010) *Communication and Interpersonal Skills in Nursing*, 2nd edn, Exeter: Learning Matters.

Balzer-Riley, J. (2004) *Communication in Nursing*, St Louis, MO: Mosby.

Benner, P. (1984) *From Novice to Expert: Excellence and Power in Clinical Nursing Practice*, Menlo Park, CA: Addison Wesley.

Callaghan, P., Playle, J., and Cooper, L. (eds) (2009) *Mental Health Nursing Skills*, Oxford: Oxford University Press.

Department of Health (2010) *Equity and Excellence: Liberating the NHS*, London: Department of Health.

Endacott, R., Jevon, P., and Cooper, L. (eds) (2009) *Clinical Nursing Skills: Core and Advanced*, Oxford: Oxford University Press.

Facebook (2011) 'Advertising data: data available by searching', available online at <http://www.facebook.com/advertising/?campaign_id=214294157440&placement=broad&creative=5811620432&keyword=advertising+facebook&extra_1=65f2e36a-7d87-83e9-caa4-000027577f68>

Foy, C. and Timmins, F. (2004) 'Improving communication in day surgery settings', *Nursing Standard*, 19(7): 37–42.

Gilbert, P. and Leahy, R. (eds) (2007) *The Therapeutic Relationship in the Cognitive Behavioural Psychotherapies*, London: Routledge.

Hargie, O. and Dickson, D. (2004) *Skilled Interpersonal Communication: Research, Theory and Practice*, London: Routledge.

Holland, K., Roxburgh, M., Johnson, M., Topping, K., Watson, R., Lauder, W., and Porter, M. (2010) 'Fitness for practice in nursing and midwifery education in Scotland, United Kingdom', *Journal of Clinical Nursing*, 19(3–4): 461–9.

Kwekkeboom, K. (1997) 'The placebo effect in symptom management', *Oncological Nursing Forum*, 24(8): 1393–9.

Learner, S. (2006) 'Fears for literacy and numeracy as new nurses fail basic tests', *Nursing Standard*, 20(49): 10.

McCabe, C. and Timmins, F. (2006) *Communication Skills for Nursing Practice*, Basingstoke: Palgrave Macmillan.

McMahon, R. (1998) 'Therapeutic nursing: theory, issues and practice', in R. McMahon and A. Pearson (eds) *Nursing as Therapy*, 2nd edn, Cheltenham: Nelson Thornes, pp. 1–25.

Miller, E. and Nambiar-Greenwood, G. (2011) 'The nurse–patient relationship', in L. Webb (ed.) *Nursing: Communication Skills in Practice*, Oxford: Oxford University Press, pp. 20–32.

Nursing and Midwifery Council (2008) *The Code: Standards of Conduct, Performance and Ethics for Nurses and Midwives*, London: NMC.

Nursing and Midwifery Council (2009) *Guidance on Professional Conduct for Nursing and Midwifery Students*, London: NMC.

Nursing and Midwifery Council (2010a) *Record Keeping: Guidance for Nurses and Midwives*, London: NMC.

Nursing and Midwifery Council (2010b) *Standards for Pre-Registration Nursing Education*, London: NMC.

Nursing and Midwifery Council (2012) 'Social networking sites', available online at <**http://www.nmc-uk.org/Nurses-and-midwives/Advice-by-topic/A/Advice/Social-networking-sites/**>

Office for National Statistics (2011) 'Internet access: households and individuals, 2011', available online at <**http://www.ons.gov.uk/ons/rel/rdit2/internet-access---households-and-individuals/2011/stb-internet-access-2011.html**>

O'Grady, L. and Jadad, A. (2010) 'Shifting from shared to collaborative decision making: a change in thinking and doing', *Journal of Participatory Medicine*, 2: e13.

Owen, A. (2004) 'The therapeutic relationship', available online at <**http://www.holisticlocal.com/articles/view/293/The+Therapeutic+Relationship**>

Pincock, S. (2004) 'Poor communication lies at heart of NHS complaints, says ombudsman', *British Medical Journal*, 328(10): 5.

Roper, N., Logan, W. W., and Tierney, A. J. (2001) *The Roper Logan Tierney Model of Nursing Based on Activities of Living*, Edinburgh: Churchill Livingstone.

Sharples, K. and Elcock, K. (2011) *Preceptorship for Newly Registered Nurses*, Exeter: Learning Matters.

Standing, M. (2010) *Clinical Judgement and Decision Making in Nursing and Inter-Professional Healthcare*, Maidenhead: Open University Press.

Thompson, C. (2003) 'Clinical experience as evidence in evidence-based practice', *Journal of Advanced Nursing*, 43(3): 230–7.

Thompson, C. and Dowding, D. (2002) *Clinical Decision Making and Judgement in Nursing*, Edinburgh: Churchill Livingstone.

Webb, L. (2011) *Nursing: Communication Skills in Practice*, Oxford: Oxford University Press.

Wosket, V. (2006) *Egan's Skilled Helper Model: Developments and Application in Counselling*, London: Routledge.

Further Reading

Burnard, P. and Gill, P. (2008) *Culture, Communication and Nursing*. Harlow: Pearson Education Ltd.

Holland, K., Jenkins, J., Soloman, J., and Whittam, S. (eds) (2008) *Applying the Roper-Logan-Tierney model in practice,* Second Edition. Edinburgh: Blackwell Science.

Useful Links and Resources

<http://www.nmc-uk.org/Documents/NMC-Publications/NMC-Record-Keeping-Guidance.pdf>

The NMC's (2010a) *Record Keeping: Guidance for Nurses and Midwives*.

<http://standards.nmc-uk.org/PublishedDocuments/Standards%20for%20pre-registration%20nursing%20education%2016082010.pdf>

The NMC's (2010b) *Standards for Pre-Registration Nursing Education*.

<http://www.ombudsman.org.uk/>

The website for the Parliamentary and Health Service Ombudsman in the UK, who oversees the complaints system.

<http://global.oup.com/uk/orc/nursing/callaghan/>

The Online Resource Centre for Callaghan et al. (2009), ch. 9 of which will help you with decision making.

<http://global.oup.com/uk/orc/nursing/endacott/>

The Online Resource Centre for Endacott et al. (2009), chs 10, 11, and 12A of which cover communication skills.

<http://global.oup.com/uk/orc/nursing/webb/>

The Online Resource Centre for Webb (2011), another book in this series, has many online resources that will help you with various aspects of communication and interpersonal skills.

7

Nursing practice and decision making

Dawn Gawthorpe

The aims of the chapter are to:

- ➔ consider what constitutes effective and appropriate decisions;
- ➔ consider decision making in acute and critical situations in all fields of practice;
- ➔ explore how nurses use a 'library' or 'bank' of experience to inform decisions;
- ➔ explore what it means to know a patient in the context of decision making;
- ➔ explore the role of intuition in nursing, and the part played by reflecting on prior knowledge and experience; and
- ➔ consider the emotive aspects of decision making in practice.

Introduction

You have already seen in earlier chapters that decision making is the cognitive process of reaching a decision—of considering a number of options from which only one can be chosen. Student nurses need to develop knowledge not only of generic nursing skills, but those related specifically to their chosen field of practice (NMC 2010). So how much knowledge do you need to be a nurse and how do you know when you have acquired it?

It is often said that 'a little knowledge is a dangerous thing'—a saying attributed to Alexander Pope (1688–1744). In nursing terms, this could mean that this small amount of knowledge can potentially mislead you into thinking that you are more competent than you actually are. How much knowledge is required to ensure competency as a qualified nurse is not easily determined, however, because we all learn in different ways and over time. Lifelong learning is advocated for all nurses and, indeed, is a requirement of continued registration (NMC 2011); as a qualified nurse, you will be making decisions on a daily basis for the rest of your working life, which will require you to be aware of best evidence for practice and patient care.

The nature of these decisions forms an important part of this chapter and there will be a number of case studies related to all fields of practice for you to consider. It is important that you do not consider and answer only those related to your own field of practice, because you might encounter a situation in which you might have to care for a child or young person on an adult ward in hospital, or during a home visit in the community: for example, a grandparent might suddenly complain of feeling unwell and collapse whilst visiting his or her grandchild on a children's ward. The Nursing and Midwifery Council (NMC) reminds us that nurses' decision making must also be shared with service users, carers, and families—that is, that we must work with people to ensure the best and most appropriate decision for their needs at that time (NMC 2010).

In order to be able to consider and attempt to answer the exercises associated with the case studies in this chapter, we need first to consider some of the issues as background knowledge.

What are effective and appropriate decisions?

How do we know what is or is not a good decision? How can we measure the quality of our decisions?

A way of undertaking this process of assessing what is an appropriate decision or not is by considering the following three stages.

1. Ask yourself: 'What will happen if I do/do not do this?' Make a list of your answers.
2. Evaluate your answers. Now consider how likely the outcomes are to occur and how serious they would be for the patient or client.
3. Develop some preventative or contingency plans—that is, consider what you could have done differently or what was already in place that may have provided you with an alternative course of action.

Another consideration here is related to how others perceive your decisions: for a decision to be considered good, then others who are involved have to believe in you and the decision that you made. The art here lies in convincing others that this was the right decision, and the best way of doing that is to be professional, be confident about your decision, and be able to explain how and why you came to make that particular decision. This is where the use of best evidence, as seen in **Chapter 3**, can make a difference.

You need to be able to tell others about the positive and negative issues associated with the decision. Nurse educators aim to engender the development of these underlying 'evidence for decision-making' skills when they ask you to participate in such learning experiences as debates, presentations, and questioning by peers, or when they undertake simulated practice in which you experience scenarios based on real clinical events and have to offer rationales for decision making. You will also have to offer rationales explaining why certain decisions were made less well.

So what is a 'bad' decision?

Some people believe that if something goes wrong, then a bad decision must have been made by the person responsible for the decision. However, as we have discussed so far, sometimes the outcomes and consequences of the decision can be unexpected and unpredictable, and none more so than those in relation to the health of the patients for whom you are caring. This is mainly because all patients are individuals with their own health backgrounds; many will have chronic health problems in which a degree of predictability can be expected, as well as patients/clients who are very knowledgeable about their symptoms and their management. The student nurse caring for the patient, however, will not necessarily be as informed and it is here that 'decision conflict' could occur. What this means is that, as a student you may feel that your decisions are governed by what the patient says; the patient may have his or her own coping strategy or way of managing his or her condition, which is not necessarily one with which you are familiar or about which you have read. This might cause some conflict in terms of your decision.

Others, of course, will have an acute health problem and, as a result, will represent a completely new experience for the patient/client and, of course, for the student nurse. Decision making in any of these situations will depend on the knowledge and skills of the student nurse at the time that a decision is required, but it must always be remembered that mentors and other qualified nurses are close by to supervise any decision-making process. (See **Chapter 5** for more on professional issues and decision making.)

Now think about a decision that you have made that has impacted on a patient in your care. When reflecting on that decision and its outcome, you have done so with different knowledge, because you will have had some feedback from your mentor about its impact and can now consider alternatives as a result. As long as the decision has been taken under supervision and caused no harm, your mentor should have asked you to consider alternatives, and to undertake some further reading and information finding.

Something that can be considered a bad decision may involve not considering *any* alternatives or choosing something that is a less-than-satisfactory alternative. Bad decisions can include choosing the wrong goal and then arriving at a poor outcome for yourself or others, or not using assessment tools to guide you in evaluating possible alternatives.

The reality is that there are really no 'bad' decisions, because hopefully, as both student and qualified nurses, we are continuously learning from those that we make and therefore developing our repertoire of skills underpinned by sound evidence-based rationale.

Action versus inaction

In the very first instance, you have to make a decision and there are options even here: do something; or do nothing. But even in choosing either to do something or to do nothing, you have made a decision.

......

 Exercise

You are talking to Mrs Gawthorpe one afternoon when she suddenly grimaces. 'Are you in pain?' you ask her.

'No', Mrs Gawthorpe replies.

You rephrase the question: 'Are you alright?'

'I just don't feel well', answers Mrs Gawthorpe. 'I can't explain it. I just feel really poorly.'

Write down what you feel you should do next.

1. Did you check Mrs Gawthorpe's physiological observations?
2. Did you call for a more senior nurse or doctor to examine Mrs Gawthorpe?

......

In relation to the first question in this exercise, even though Mrs Gawthorpe's observations are not due to be recorded, you may have undertaken an assessment of her haemodynamic state—blood pressure, pulse, temperature, and respiratory rate and oxygen saturation monitoring—but nothing in the results may have given you cause for concern. *Why did you do decide to do this?*

One of the reasons for your action is that you require knowledge to make a decision and you were looking for physiological clues that something may be wrong that has not, as yet, manifested itself in particular signs or symptoms.

In relation to the second question, you may also have decided on another option of calling a more senior nurse or the doctor, and asking him or her: 'Will you just check Mrs Gawthorpe for me?'

Often, we make this decision because we cannot find the answers on which to base our decisions and that, in part, is because of the limited experience that we may have had to date; so the more junior you are, the more likely you are to welcome others making these decisions. Actually calling for assistance is allowing you to develop skills in meeting Domain 2, Competency 7.1, of the NMC *Standards for Pre-Registration Nursing Education* (NMC 2010), which requires, for example as an adult nurse, that you are able 'to recognize early signs of illness through accurate assessments'. What you, as a qualified nurse, did was complete a very basic assessment of the patient. For the more senior nurse, a tachycardia and hypotension with an irregular respiratory rate may indicate a patient in shock, accompanied with a hyperpyrexia, and the qualified experienced nurse may consider that the patient could well have a much more serious underlying problem.

Who is actually making the decision for whom?

When we use words such as 'morals' and 'ethics', most of us think about things that we have read in the newspaper or considered in a classroom session, and often they are related to topics such as end-of-life decisions, abortion, and resources. 'Morals' are defined by Griffith and Tengnah (2010) as what a person believes is right. Moral dilemmas arise when there are choices to be made—when we are faced with two options and we do not consider either to be entirely satisfactory.

Activity

Two patients ask for a bedpan at the same time.

1. Who gets it first: the patient nearest the sluice; the patient who looks the most desperate; or the patient who you personally like the most?
2. What would your decision have been in relation to the two patients and who should get a bed pan first?
3. Consider what the main difficulties were in trying to make a decision.

Another problem here is that it can also be difficult to predict what the outcomes may be concerning the decision that you make. Knowing about the subject of ethics is important and it can help you to support the achievement of the decision-making process, but not necessarily the outcome. It can be argued that every decision that we make is based on a moral or ethical principle.

Consider the following scenario and possible optional decisions.

Case study 7.1

Mr Singh, aged 46, has been diagnosed with a malignant cerebral tumour, which is expected to be life-limiting. The oncologist has discussed a number of treatment options with Mr Singh, who now has a decision to make. He asks you which treatment option he should choose.

(Continued)

Case study 7.1 (Continued)

Question

How will you approach this decision?

Issues to consider

In deciding what to do, you may well refer to tools for decision making, some of which were discussed in **Chapter 1**, taking into account the four-principle approach of ethical decision making, as advocated by Beauchamp and Childress (2001), which includes consideration of respect for autonomy, non-maleficence, beneficence, and justice. You would also consider the NMC's *The Code: Standards of Conduct, Performance and Ethics for Nurses and Midwives* (NMC 2008), which offers you professional guidance in relation to the care of patients such as Mr Singh.

What is important, however, is to recognize that the patient needs you to help him understand why he is being asked to make a decision and your role here is to facilitate this process. The decision is whether you undertake this role yourself or feel that another staff member may be more suitable—perhaps Mr Singh's named nurse, who has known him for several weeks rather than an agency nurse who is meeting him for the first time.

You may wish to develop a checklist of points to consider when deciding what might be the most ethical response, such as the following.

1. 'Does this choice fit with my own professional and personal values?'
2. 'What are the likely decision conflicts that might arise?'
3. 'Where is the evidence and did I consider it in a logical sequence rather than simply choose the first alternative?'
4. 'Did I jump to my own conclusion? If I did, did I use any previous experience?'
5. 'Can I implement my decision?' (This part of the process gets you to think about your accountability.)

Using a similar framework to that outlined in **Case study 7.1** can improve personal satisfaction, help you to offer better patient care, and help to ensure that you promote the best interest of your patient.

Making decisions in acute and critical care situations

An increase in knowledge will be gained from observing, participating, and experiencing clinical practice within both generic and field-specific placements. Most of what is learned also helps you to develop your technical skills. Past experiences, including learning in previous placements, help to guide our actions.

Reflective Activity

Decisions in communication and being a student nurse

Think about your very first clinical placement. What knowledge and skills did you think you brought with you? For some of you, you came straight from school or college, and you may not feel as though you knew very much about nursing and that you did not bring any skills with you.

Think about the first patient you met. What did you do first and why? Did you introduce yourself? If you answered 'yes', then how and why did you do this? Did you just say 'Hello Mr/Mrs ...'? Or did you follow on with 'My name is ... and I'm a first-year student'? What were you intending to do when you introduced yourself?

Write your answers down in your learning diary.

 Top Tips

It is always good practice, as part of your placement learning, to have a book of some kind in which you can write down reflections, make notes about various types of condition or health problem that you encounter as a reminder to read up on them in textbooks, to find evidence to support the care given, or to discover the different types of medication and their side effects. In this way, you will begin to build up a 'bank' or 'learning library' of knowledge for future practice, and also reaffirm your current knowledge and skills in caring for different patients who may have a range of illnesses, or with whom you work in encouraging self-care and decision making in maintaining health and well-being. Do remember to anonymize any events to ensure that confidentiality is maintained.

Consider the situation in **Case study 7.2**.

The following four case studies ask you to consider how your decisions can vary depending on the situation in which you find yourself or the point at which you are in your nursing education programme.

Case study 7.2 Decisions in prioritizing care

You have just started your early shift and you have been assigned to work in a different bay from the one to which you are used. The bay in which you are working has five female patients (each one has agreed to being called by their first name):

● Annie is aged 92 and has been a patient for two weeks;

● Meryl was admitted that morning for investigations and is expected only to be an in-patient for the day;

● Karishma, Bridget, and Lai Chi are due to be discharged later today.

At this point during the shift, you have served the breakfasts, during which three of the women were very chatty and pleased to see you. Karishma, however, did not join in the conversation, instead sitting quietly, and does not make eye contact either with the other women or you.

The next task is to prioritize the care for the rest of the shift.

Question

To which of the patients do you decide to go first?

Issues to consider

If you go to Karishma, then you may well end up spending longer with her, trying to ascertain why she seems quiet and withdrawn. You may have recognized that there is a lot of pressure on your time, including making sure that Meryl gets to the right department to have her investigations completed in a timely manner, and getting the discharge letters and prescriptions ready for Bridget and Lai Chi.

All of this activity allows you to get the tasks of the day done—but what demonstrates caring?

For some nurses, it will be easier to determine which patients can articulate what they require, to deal with them swiftly and straightforwardly, and then to give time to Karishma, because they recognize that she may need more of their time. The problem with this is how others might perceive the nurse in this situation: they might think that the nurse is avoiding work.

Here is the dilemma: there are no easy answers, but what is important for you as the nurse is to recognize this and to understand why you choose to go to one patient first rather than another. So what would be an appropriate decision here? Write down your answer so that you can return to it later.

The best decision would be to recognize this dilemma and to ask for some help in trying to deal with more than one situation at a time. It is important also to recognize

(Continued)

Case study 7.2 (Continued)

the contribution of those who do assist you. (You are encouraged to read Cox, C. (2012) 'Caring: a patient's perspective', *Gastrointestinal Nursing*, 10(2): 5, an editorial in which a nurse gives a very succinct account of caring from the perspective of her own experience of being a patient.)

Next, let us consider the settings in which we may make decisions, and the challenges and skills with which this presents us.

Case study 7.3 Decisions in therapeutic practice

Danny Bisto is a 66-year-old man with a diagnosis of paranoid schizophrenia, who has, over the past twenty years, been cared for in and by a number of mental health services and professionals. You meet him for the first time while in the final week of a community mental health placement. Your mentor has been accompanying you and, for this week, has asked you (under supervision) to take the lead in caring for the clients to help you to develop your management skills. Danny has been on antipsychotic therapy for a number of years, but calls his community nurse to say that he is being eaten alive and can she come with the pest team. The community nurse is concerned, because she reports that Danny's condition has been very stable for the past year, and she arranges to visit him that day.

When you arrive at the house, Danny asks you to help him to get comfortable in his chair, saying that he cannot breathe too well because the dust mites are eating away at his lungs and they are going to burrow through his skin.

Question

How do you as the nurse decide what to do next?

Issues to consider

There is quite a complex series of decisions that take place here, especially if this is the first client contact that you have ever had. Questions that you may ask yourself include the following.

(Continued)

Case study 7.3 (Continued)

- 'Is what Mr Bisto is claiming the truth?'
- 'Is this client considered still to be acutely ill in terms of his mental health?'
- 'Does he, in fact, have any breathing problems at all?'
- 'Can I do this?'
- 'Should I be doing this?'
- 'Do I need help to do this?'
- 'What does Mr Bisto mean by "comfortable"? Is it helping him to sit up or rearrange the cushions, or will he ask me to do something about which I know nothing?'

What is important in this exercise is the information that you were given before you met the patient and that you, as the nurse, should keep monitoring the situation. In the first instance, instinct or intuition might tell you not to do anything other than plump up the cushions—but when he says that this is no better, you need to continue this monitoring activity. You need to assess the patient's breathing before doing anything else— remember: look, listen, and feel. Is the patient exhibiting signs of respiratory distress?

You need to be able to decide if this client's condition is stable or deteriorating; then you can move on to exploring what he is saying and have a look at his skin to see if there is any evidence of rashes or scratching, which may indicate that something is causing skin irritation. It is very important here to get the client to describe what is happening, because verbal cues are useful in deciding what to do next.

An important issue here is that you are not alone: you have a mentor who has known the patient for a long time and one of the best decisions that you may need to make is to ask for her help.

Case study 7.3 is an example of an instance in which you, as the student nurse, must recognize your limitations, not least because The NMC Code (NMC 2008) and *The Prep Handbook* (NMC 2011) require you to recognize and work within the limits of your competence.

Case study 7.4 Decision making and knowing that something is wrong

The nurse is observing Jin, a 12-year-old boy admitted to the surgical ward following an appendectomy. The post-operative notes indicate that physiological measurements should be undertaken half-hourly and the wound checked hourly.

The nurse has been looking after the patient for two hours now and the observations have been within acceptable parameters. The nurse is walking past the patient, who appears to be breathing quite noisily—snoring in fact—but the observations are not due for another 20 minutes. The patient may well be sleeping or it might be the effects of the analgesia—but something makes the nurse go to the patient and try to rouse him.

Questions

1. What do you think led the nurse to make this decision?
2. What are the implications of this action?
3. What could be the implications of no action?
4. What other decisions do you think that the nurse could have made?

Issues to consider

The nurse may have used intuition as a guide to take action and try to rouse the patient. Scientific knowledge may have been used in terms of noisy breathing acting as an alert that there may have been a change in levels of consciousness impelling the nurse to take action. Taking action to try to rouse the patient enables the nurse to confirm or refute suspicions regarding Jin's recovery from the surgery. Taking no action might result in undetected physiological changes including altered levels of consciousness. The nurse, we remember, is accountable for actions and omissions.

Activity

Make notes of your answers to all of the questions in these case studies, and discuss all of your decisions and (hypothetical) actions with your mentor. Doing so will help you to work towards achieving the competencies that are the focus of this chapter—namely, 'Nursing practice and decision making' (NMC 2010).

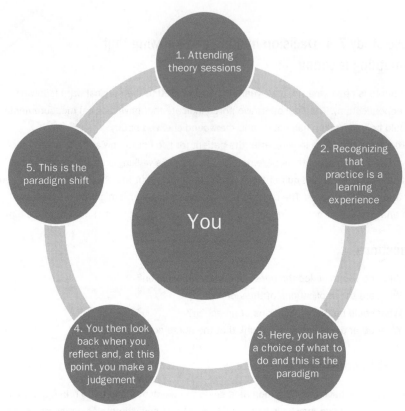

Figure 7.1 Developing new ways of thinking for decision making.

What is initially important is that we understand this way of thinking about nursing practice (often called a 'paradigm'): that is, 'this is the way that something works' or simply that 'this is the way it is'. The next important skill is to recognize that these paradigms, or ways of thinking and believing, about nursing practice can shift and that, as a student, it is essential, in order to learn new knowledge and skills, that you should always be open to new learning experiences.

Figure 7.1 may help you to consider how a nurse may become part of this so called 'paradigm shift'. This is, of course, a very simplistic use and explanation of paradigms and how they apply to changes in how you make decisions over time. (See the 'Further reading' listed at the end of this chapter for more on this.)

Case study 7.5 Using reflection to develop clinical skills

Imagine that Nurse Brack is reflecting on his clinical skills development in relation to giving a patient an injection. Using **Figure 7.1** as a guide, Nurse Brack thinks about the first time he gave a patient an injection.

Stage 1 Attending the theory sessions

We had a clinical skills session in which we practised on false muscle specimens. I was nervous because that was just fun and we still have to do this on real patients. I went away and read my notes over and over again, to try to remember the different types of injection and injection sites. I'll *never* be able to remember them all.

Stage 2 Recognizing that practice is a learning experience

Patients come in all shapes and sizes. It's alright saying 'into this muscle'—but what do we do with a patient with wasted muscles? I need to find out.

Stage 3 The initial 'paradigm' (Nurse Brack's way of thinking about giving an injection)

Nurse Brack now has a choice: he can refrain from the practice experience because he is nervous, or he can seize the valuable learning opportunity while having the support of other nurses or mentors.

I thought to myself 'I can do this', because I'm learning to be a nurse and know that it's better to get this over and done with as soon as possible—like a big hurdle. That's what I think, anyway, so 'best get on with it' I thought. My mentor was helpful, but she did have a different way of doing this injection. I think she just knew the patient a bit better than I did.

Stage 4 Changing ways of thinking about the giving of injections

Nurse Brack undertakes his first injection on a patient and looks back at the learning experience. Here is where the paradigm shift occurs, because he recognizes that there are alternatives, and he therefore changes his ideas and his beliefs about what he already thinks. He recognizes the need to adapt what he is doing for this patient, based on all of the learning that has taken place.

I thought I knew how to give this injection and that every patient was given it in the same way. But it became clear that my mentor was right and that, when you get to know your patients, it's important to consider not just the 'doing' of giving the injection, but

(Continued)

Case study 7.5 (Continued)

also to think about the patient as an individual each time. I had to adapt and make a different decision the next time I gave an injection to a patient, who was a young man who'd had his leg amputated after an accident. My first every patient had been an elderly gentleman, who was an insulin-dependent diabetic.

Stage 5 The new way of thinking about making decisions

The 'paradigm shift', or shift in Nurse Brack's way of thinking about nursing practice, has taken place. Eventually, we not only know *how*, but also *why* we are doing something—in this case study, giving an injection—but as a result of a change in thinking through learning about different ways of nursing, we are consequently able to consider appropriately each patient's individual requirements.

These four case studies through which you have worked will help you to develop generic skills and to meet the requirement that you 'must be able to recognize and respond to the needs of all people who come into [your] care' (NMC 2010).

In the next section of this chapter, we can consider other ways in which to gain this clinical or professional knowledge to inform our decision making. Sometimes, we use the term 'library of experience', or a 'bank' of experiences, from which we can pick and choose both theoretical and practical experiences to inform our decisions. These decisions do not necessarily require a major change in the way in which we think about something or what we believe something to be; rather, these types of decision are those in which we already have this 'library full of experiences and knowledge and skills already there'. We simply have to sort them out, and then choose the best and most appropriate ones to use in different situations.

It is important to remember that this learning to make decisions is not dependent on what we already know in the 'library', but that we make new additions on an ongoing basis throughout our nursing careers. It is this ability and the need to do this that ensures that we become 'expert' practitioners, as defined by Benner (1984).

Using a 'library' (or 'bank') of experience

Gaining this knowledge involves the application of our memory, but also involves allowing the brain to do what it needs to do—that is, to *think*. We need to be able to think: we need to have knowledge about a subject, but certainly in nursing we need to be able to *apply* this to an enormous variety of seen, but mainly unseen, situations. We need to be able not only to make decisions appropriately, but also to problem solve.

> ## Activity
>
> A nurse, for example, may be problem solving when a patient expresses that the chest pain she is experiencing feels different from that which she felt in the morning.
>
> Write down what you think the nurse may be thinking and compare it to the suggestions that follow.

There and then, the nurse thinks the following.

- 'What shall I do first?'
- 'What do I think may be happening to the patient?'
- 'What are the potential consequences of leaving this patient to attend to another?'
- 'Which of the above options should I choose?'
- 'Whichever option I choose, can I get others to help me?'

So, let us think about the various options. Before we do this, however, consider the next exercise, which has been attributed to John Adair (2007).

⊕ Exercise

Here is a pattern of dots:

```
.   .   .

.   .   .

.   .   .
```

Now try to connect the dots using *four* consecutive lines (without taking your pen or pencil off the paper).

Let us think about what you were doing as you tried to complete this 'dot' puzzle.

Adair (2007) suggests that you were 'analysing', 'synthesizing', 'imagining', and 'valuing':

- The **analysis** occurs when you separate a whole into component parts—so, in relation to this exercise, you might question what you are being asked to do.
- **Synthesis** involves putting things together to make a whole—for example, if I give you a pile of building blocks and ask you to make a tower.
- It is likely that you will **imagine** how it might look in the first instance and then stack the building blocks one on top of another.
- Finally, **valuing** has many meanings, such as giving consideration to whether the task was successful and making comment about the process.

If you now consider what you did to achieve the set task in this exercise, did you ask yourself a number of questions first?

We refer to this as a 'question sequence' and **Figure 7.2** demonstrates what is involved.

The belief of behaviourist Isobel Briggs Myers (1897–1980) was that a person's decision-making process depends on his or her cognitive style—that is, the way in which he or she thinks, understands, and remembers information. In 1962, she devised the Myers-Briggs Type Indicator (MBTI), which is now used by many organizations, for example, to determine how employees make decisions and which of them is the best at doing this. Her writings were updated in 2000 (Briggs Myers 2000).

This tool looks at two cognitive functions: those that are 'rational'—so thinking and feeling—and those that are 'irrational'—that is, sensing and intuition. There are four scoring sections:

- thinking and feeling;
- extroversion and introversion;

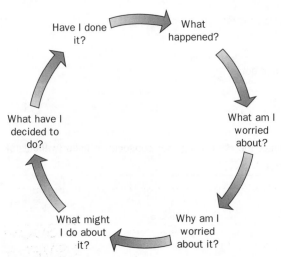

Figure 7.2 Question sequence.

- judgement and perception; and
- sensing and intuition.

You may well already know your cognitive style, but if not, visit **<http://www.myers-briggs.org/>** to read more about the MBTI. This information may give you an insight into the way in which you and others make decisions.

Developing this library of experience within a nursing programme

Let us now consider how you use a 'library of experience' within your practice as a student nurse.

....

 Exercise

Imagine that, under supervision, you have been asked to look after a ten-bedded bay of patients for the whole of an early shift to help you to develop managerial skills. List the resources that will be available to you. Now identify which year of study you are in and compare your answers with those of some other student nurses who may be in clinical practice with you.

....

You may have considered the following:

- (first-year student) other staff, mentors, auxiliaries, support workers, other students;
- (second-year student) all of the above, plus ward clerks, pharmacists, relatives, own knowledge to date; and
- (third-year student) all of the above plus more consideration of the environmental influences, admissions, discharges, whether there are enough medicines and linen, whether the meals have been ordered for the patients, whether there is an operating list and, if so, which patient is first, and whether the pre-operative checklist has been completed.

This should not be an exhaustive list; indeed, you may have considered other things as well.

If you were to consider what types of decision you might have to make during the day, you may list:

- what to do first or how to prioritize care based on the information given in handover;
- how to allocate staff;
- what task to delegate to whom;
- assessing and then reassessing patients;

- how to time-manage;
- whether you need more information; and
- whether to change any plans that you initially made.

Recognizing that there are differences in making decisions for and in nursing

All nursing programmes, in whatever university and partner health care organizations you are studying (and in different countries as well), aim to prepare students to learn what types of decision nurses have to make—starting in the first year, through to becoming the student nurse who is prepared to start making decisions in the final year and who is ready for the transition to registrant. (Further development of these ideas can be found in **Chapter 13**.)

In the new NMC Standards (NMC 2010), this escalation of skills development is engendered by means of the progression criteria for each year of a three-year programme (and by meeting the required 4,600 hours of learning in theory and practice). For Progression points 1 and 2, for example, students are expected to consider the safety and protection of people of all ages, whilst demonstrating the professional values, attitudes, and behaviours that are expected of a nurse. Progression point 2 also expects nurse educators to develop programmes of study that allow the nursing student to show that he or she can work more independently, and to demonstrate his or her ability to work as an autonomous practitioner by the time of registration.

Another way in which we acquire knowledge to help us to make decisions within nursing is through our clinical practice. Professor Patricia Benner from the University of California introduced us to the evidence that nurses acquire skills and an understanding of nursing care through both knowledge gained from a theoretical perspective, as well as the variety of experiences to which nurses are exposed in practice. In her book *From Novice to Expert*, Benner (1984) identified that most of us can come to 'know how', for example, to undertake the task of manual blood pressure recording, but that nurses particularly need to also develop the 'know that'.

Using this example, anyone can be taught how ('knowing how') to take a manual blood pressure recording, but an understanding that a reading of a diastolic pressure higher than 100 mmHg needs further intervention is part of the 'knowing that'.

In her research, Benner (1984) identified five stages to skills acquisition: novice; advanced beginner; becoming competent; being proficient; and, finally, expert.

Table 7.1 briefly summarizes these stages and their meaning, with reference to how we can consider Benner's (1984) work and findings in the context of a student nurse. It is important to note that these stages were applied to qualified nurses but that they could be applied in part to the student level prior to that transition to becoming a qualified 'Novice' nurse.

Table 7.1 Benner's novice-to-expert stages and the possible explanation as applied to the student nurse and qualified nurse

Novice	The nursing student usually has little or no background experience, and will often find it difficult to discern between what is relevant and irrelevant in a given situation.
Advanced beginner	The nursing student has experience of actual incidents, and can recall and remember important components, which can guide his or her actions.
Competent	The nursing student can hopefully recognize patterns, and has the ability to decide which facets of a situation need attention and what can be ignored. The student may follow rules or guidelines, but can also devise new ways of working through reasoning. Usually, the student has been practising for two or three years at this point.
Proficient	The qualified nurse looks at the whole situation and draws on a wide range of background knowledge, appearing to have an intuitive understanding of a situation.
Expert	The expert nurse does not need rules, guidelines, and principles to help her to understand a situation and to respond in an appropriate manner, because of his or her wide range of experience. The expert nurse is able to hone in on the problem, without being distracted and spending too much time on other options. The expert nurse also demonstrates an intuitive grasp of situations.

Source: Possible outcomes of different Stages (Interpreted from Benner 1984)

So, how do you, as a student, develop these skills, especially in relation to making decisions? One of the most important ways is by using past experience (and the library of knowledge) and also three other approaches:

- developing checklists;
- reflecting back on critical incidents; and
- listing ideas that have worked previously.

In this way, you can develop a repertoire of responses that can be applied in any clinical situation.

Work conducted by Greenhalgh (2002) suggests that novices adhere to plans or rules. Knowledge gained at this stage can be scientific, for example in considering **Case study 7.4**, the student will need to have an understanding of the relevant anatomy and physiology of the respiratory and cardiovascular system to understand and interpret the signs and symptoms with which the patient presents. Those further along in their programme, who are becoming competent, begin to see the longer-term picture and goals, recognizing when there is a need to make decisions and then actually making them.

You may have participated in decision-making exercises within a classroom situation, giving you the opportunity to rehearse what you may or may not decide to do. Increasingly, you may be asked to consider a patient with more complex care needs to develop these skills.

Registered nurses who are considered to be what Benner (1984) terms 'expert' practitioners often do not rely on guidelines and rules; rather, they utilize this intuitive skill on a regular basis. (See **Chapter 1** for more on intuitive decision making.)

If you are a third-year student and we look back to your nursing practice in the first year, it might have been inconceivable that you would be making the decisions that you are now undertaking. A third-year nursing student, however, can draw on the knowledge and skills that he or she has accumulated from previous placements—that is, from his or her 'library'.

So now what you need to do is to reflect on what you did and why.

Let us consider this in the context of a familiar hospital situation, for all fields of practice learning.

Activity

What are the benefits of a handover? Consider this question in the context of what you may know or have experienced yourself about handovers.

A handover, for example, should afford the team the opportunity to ask questions and to clarify anything before the previous shift leaves. You may wish to read the findings of Pothier et al. (2005) and Currie (2002) on this practice of handover.

It is also important to remember the part that patients have in this now traditionally named nursing practice. In fact, they are central to its purpose. You need to go and talk to the patients as soon as possible when you have been given information about them at the handover, and find out how they are feeling and whether information given to you about their well-being and health status still holds true. This will also give you the opportunity to check for non-verbal cues, as well as verbal ones, and help you to decide which patients require priority care. Making decisions about patient care when you have neither talked to nor seen the patient, especially if you need to delegate some responsibilities, is not recommended as good practice, especially if you are accountable and responsible for his or her care. Actually visiting with the patients soon after handover helps with the delegation of staff. Whilst most of the team will either have been allocated to a bay or group of patients, this might need changing, depending on the condition or health status of certain patients.

How do we know, then, when we talk to and observe patients, what decisions to make? One way, as discussed in **Chapter 1**, is through intuitive knowledge and the important issue discussed in **Chapter 4**—that is, reflecting on prior knowledge and experience.

Exploring the role of intuition in nursing, and the part played by reflecting on prior knowledge and experience

Intuition is often considered to be a characteristic of expertise. For example, you may wonder how the charge nurse knows that the patient's condition is deteriorating. When you stand there as a student nurse and observe his or her assessment, it will appear almost magical, as well as difficult to explain. When you ask the charge nurse how he or she knew, he or she is likely to use terms such as 'gut feeling', 'instinct', and 'second nature'.

The intuitive model of decision making was discussed in **Chapter 1** and you should revisit this chapter if you need a reminder, so that you will understand what is being discussed here. Parahoo (2006) suggests that intuitive decision making is also about knowing and behaving that is not based on rational reasoning. Put another way, we could look at it as knowing, but without knowing how we know. We sometimes refer to this as our 'sixth sense' or others may call this an 'inner voice', 'having a hunch', or even 'wisdom'.

Think back to when you were younger and were about to cross for the first time a busy road that you did not know. Could you hear that inner voice telling you to stop, look, and listen before you thought about stepping off the pavement? Did you waver for just one second to be truly sure that no cars were coming? In fact, most of us still do this as something that is inherent in our behaviour as adults, if we have been taught this practice and if we have continued to do this ever since that time.

As nurses, we make informed decisions that affect the lives of our patients (service users). Alison Gadsby (2008), writing in the *Nursing Times*, said that she believed that she had a natural nursing instinct and that whilst evidence-based practice was important, the ability to use and trust his or her own instincts is what makes a good nurse into a great one.

Instinct, arguably, cannot be taught. A frequent question that a nursing student on placement will find himself or herself asking a mentor or colleagues is: 'How did you know that would happen?'

If you read about intuition, then there is often a discussion about what the characteristics or features of it are and how it is recognized. Phrases often used include 'something done automatically', or 'it is an emotional response'. Those nurses using intuition in their decision making cannot normally recognize what processes are involved. They often have a very quick perception of what is occurring, whilst you may be still trying to make sense of the situation. They often do not only deal with the problem-solving element, but also consider the consequences. At times, intuition seems to make the difference between life and death (see **Chapter 1**).

Here is a case study for you to consider from my own experience as a nurse.

Case study 7.6

An unknown man (no name is available), around 6 foot or 1.8 metres tall, is transferred from the referring hospital after being stabilized following a traumatic brain injury caused by a road traffic accident in which he was hit by a car. The patient is unconscious,

(Continued)

Case study 7.6 (Continued)

intubated, and ventilated. As part of the nursing handover, the accompanying nurse reports about a wound that the patient has to the mid-thigh region: 'I've cleaned it and it doesn't look too bad.'

Question

What will you do in response to this statement? Write your answer in your learning diary.

Issues to consider

The decisions that I made in this situation were as follows. For me, as the nurse accepting the patient, assessing the wound was not an immediate priority—unlike the safe transfer of the patient from a temporary ventilator to a permanent one, and undertaking a neurological assessment to establish if there had been any deviation from the base-line assessment that the transferring nurse had completed.

My decision was influenced by the knowledge that I had of undertaking both primary and secondary surveys, which I had learned some ten years previously as a student nurse working in an accident and emergency (A&E) department. However, rather than simply dismiss this information, I had an obligation to go back and examine the wound for myself. I had accepted responsibility and a duty of care to the patient.

The information that the nurse gave me was that the wound was a very clean symmetrical wound—that something has sliced the skin cleanly and that it was not very bloody or swollen.

In order to decide what to do next, I had to remember from the clinical skills sessions that I had undertaken what types of wound there were and how they may be caused, given that the patient was hit by a vehicle.

I was concerned that we were missing something significant.

The clues were not only what the nurse said, but what she did *not* say. The things that I was expecting her to comment on included blood loss and swelling. My decision was to bring my concerns to the attention of the medical staff, as a consequence of which the leg was X-rayed and it was found that the patient had a fractured femur, with associated internal bleeding.

Was this intuition? On reflection, I think that, in this case, based on the fact that some believe intuitive judgements to be based on visual and verbal cues, it was what happened on this occasion. Given that the patient was critically ill, this wound was remarkably clean and not bleeding at all, which made me suspicious. This suspicion was based on the fact that I expected this wound to be oozing and so surmised that if this was not apparent externally, then perhaps it was occurring internally.

(Continued)

Case study 7.6 (Continued)

If we think back to some of the other exercises in this chapter, this is what you have been doing: looking for these clues. Put simply, you were trying to get the jigsaw pieces to fit together, so that you could see the picture clearly. You may well recognize that you used something akin to Adair's (2007) questioning sequence, in which he asks the reader to 'think': think about any number of possibilities, no matter how obscure; work though the probabilities; engage others to do the same and, between all of you, you will probably recognize what the next course of action should be—and a decision will be made.

One of the next decisions to be made was to find out more about the patient.

We used the patient's clothing to give us some very valuable information. The unknown patient had been wearing a scout uniform. The Scout Association has members aged between 5 and 26, but most scouts are aged between 10 and 18. How did I know this? I and other staff members had recognized the uniform, because we had children who had been scouts.

Here was a group of adult nurses working in A&E, thinking that they were caring for an adult, but potentially we were caring for a young person. His height, as well, had added to our thinking that this patient was a young adult. The decision here involved whether we needed to involve paediatric services.

What students in any field of practice need to develop are the skills of listening to the sound of intuition—that is, the ability to recognize that quiet inner voice that is telling you that something is 'not right' about a patient. You then need to be confident to rely on your intuition, not excluding all of the available evidence and facts that are presented to you, but also weighing these up before selecting from the presented alternatives. Look for the clues and cues that intuition gives you, and follow them through. Finally, you need to let your intuition lead you to action. It might be that your intuition makes connections that others cannot readily see, but this can often lead you to more choices and alternatives.

Let us continue to consider the situation of this young man—this time, hypothetically.

He is now three days post extubation and you, as a student nurse in placement on that ward, are asked to carry out a neurological assessment under supervision using the Glasgow Coma scale.

The difficulty with which you are faced is that whilst the patient is answering all of your questions related to time, place, and person, the answers are consistently incorrect. It would be easy to put this down to the traumatic brain injury that the patient has experienced as a result of his accident, but intuition tells you that you must check with his parents that he did not have a communication problem prior to the accident. Had the patient been conscious on admission, the nurse would have asked the patient questions directly, but this part of the patient's journey did not occur in the usual way.

(Continued)

Case study 7.6 (Continued)

It may well be that this young man has a known learning difficulty, which, given that he is in an adult environment, may not necessarily feature on an admission checklist. The reason why you should ask his parents about communication is that you will want to be sure that you can communicate with him in the most appropriate way and that you have not made any assumptions about him or his health status at the time. Why? Simply put, years of experience tell me that we must try to identify a 'base line' of knowledge about our patient and whether there is any deviation from that base-line assessment.

Case study 7.6 may appear to some of you as being very 'adult nursing' focused and, in some aspects, it is with regards to the clinical placement in which some students would have met the patient.

However, this scenario could be used to explain similar examples from any field-of-practice situation, because when a person is unconscious with no apparent information about him or her, we cannot assume anything about that patient as an individual, nor can we categorize him or her as an 'adult nursing' patient or a 'mental health' nursing patient. Of course, if the patient had been a child clearly around the age of 6, we would have been able to make a clear judgement that the child would be cared for by children's nurses after being in A&E. The parents, however, are adults and, as such, children's nurses have to know how to work with them in the care of the child, and must have the knowledge and skills to understand adult behaviour and needs. This is why the NMC Standards (NMC 2010) now include a set of generic competencies that apply to *all* fields of practice learning, as well as the more field-specific ones.

Dealing with the outcomes of decision making in nursing practice

Most decisions involve an element of risk. The future is never absolutely certain and so we choose from a series of alternatives. According to Joseph-Williams et al. (2010), regret is the second most cited emotion after anxiety. A common goal of all decisions is that we try to reduce any potential for regret. People choose between alternative courses of action, or between action and inaction. When we make our decision, we do so based on what might be the most appropriate course of action and employ words such as 'probable' and 'likely'.

So for example, Mrs Gawthorpe, whom we met in the first exercise, says that she is in pain following her appendicectomy yesterday. You may wonder whether she can have some analgesia or whether we should even give her analgesia. The choices are 'Yes' or 'No', and are dependent on your status as either a student nurse, a registrant or qualified nurse, or a nurse who can prescribe medication. Often, indecisiveness is because there are a number of obstacles in the way, of which the following are some of the most common.

- *Not understanding your role in a given situation*—For example, as a student nurse, your patient has collapsed and the emergency team commences cardiopulmonary resuscitation (CPR), but you are unsure whether you should offer to carry on chest compression or not. When would be an appropriate time?
- *A lack of motivation*
- *Uncertainty* is relevant to decision making because it is about the future and we all know that the future is never absolutely certain. Uncertainty is about making choices between alternatives and there is nearly always uncertainty about what would be the best choice. Sometimes, we simply guess what might be the best course of action.

  However, we could develop skills to reduce the level of guesswork, so we need to look at probability, which means that, as nurses, we need to have an understanding of statistics—that is, we need to develop our numeracy skills in order to analyse statistical data. Probability has two facets: one is objective, which lets us look at how often something will occur based on statistical analysis; the other is subjective and starts with an opinion such as what is your view of this occurring. Some risks faced by our patients are so great that there can be no real alternative.
- Some decisions we make will lead to *regret*, especially those in which there is no clearly preferred option. For example, suppose that a patient has cancer: should he or she have chemotherapy or radiotherapy with all of its known and unknown side effects, or should he or she choose not to undergo further treatment? Whilst undergoing further treatment may prolong his or her life, the patient's quality of life may be affected—but doing nothing may hasten the dying process. Neither option appears preferable and yet a decision is required.
- *Fearing past mistakes*—Sometimes, the risks are so great that we can feel there are no real alternatives. An example might be that, whilst reducing staff ratio on a ward may be a safe decision, it will not be considered a safe decision in the future if it risks the patient experience and if patient safety deteriorates, which could lead to an increase in critical incidents and complaints.

  The caveat 'if it can go wrong it will go wrong', whilst pessimistic, is realistic. It allows us to use anticipation when we consider alternatives. Working in nursing means working in a world of uncertainty—a patient's condition can change at any moment—and one thing associated with a good decision is trying to anticipate adverse consequences. We could spend an inordinate time worrying about past decisions, the so-called 'fearing the worst', but we need to look forward and consider the possible consequences, because doing so will increase our ability to deal with regret.

Conclusion

Clinical decision making is a skill that nursing students learn gradually through caring for patients and observing how those who support them in practice make decisions. Nothing can be a substitute for actually taking the time to talk to, and question and observe, patients and clients on a regular basis. As a student, you need to take every opportunity to be involved in decision-making processes and to develop your own 'library of experiences'. Alongside this, nursing students need to develop underpinning theoretical knowledge and any evidence that could support the decision-making process and outcomes.

An understanding of decision-making frameworks can help to ensure that professional, legal, and ethical aspects are addressed and that the patient's interest remains uppermost. The issues discussed in this chapter apply to all fields of practice in relation to the NMC Standards (NMC 2010) and the third domain, 'Nursing practice and decision making'. In **Part 3**, the issues discussed in the chapters comprising both **Parts 1** and **2**, such as this one, will be applied and considered in relation to each of the four fields-of-practice knowledge and skills in each of the four domains. Decision making is central to nursing practice in any context, and it is anticipated that the case studies and discussion points in this chapter will support your development of the key skills and knowledge to achieve the competencies that you require to become a registered nurse.

References

Adair, J. (2007) *Decision-Making and Problem-Solving Strategies*, London and Philadelphia, PA: Kogan Page.

Beauchamp, T. L. and Childress, J. F. (2001) *Principles of Biomedical Ethics*, 5th edn, Oxford and New York: Oxford University Press.

Benner, P. (1984) *From Novice to Expert: Excellence and Power in Clinical Nursing Practice*, Menlo Park, CA: Addison Wesley.

Benner, P., Tanner, C. A., and Chesla, C. A. (1996) *Expertise in Nursing Practice: Caring, Clinical Judgment and Ethics*, New York: Springer.

Briggs Myers, I. (2000) *An Introduction to Type: A Guide to Understanding Your Results on the Myers-Briggs Type Indicator*, 6th edn, Oxford: Oxford Psychologists Press.

Caldon, L. J., Collins, K. A., Reed, M. W., and Sivell, S. (2010) 'Clinicians' concerns about decision support interventions for patients facing breast cancer surgery options: understanding the challenge of implementing shared decision making', *Health Expectations*, 14(2): 133–46.

Cox, C. (2012) 'Caring: a patient's perspective', *Gastrointestinal Nursing*, 10(2): 5.

Currie, J. (2002) 'Improving the efficiency of patient handover', *Emergency Nurse*, 10(3): 24–8.

Gadsby, A. (2008) 'Opinion: intuition is the common element across nursing', *Nursing Times*, 13 February, available online at <http://www.nursingtimes.net/alison-gadsby-intuition-is-the-common-element-across-nursing/701726.article>

Greenhalgh, T. (2002) 'Uneasy bedfellows reconciling intuition and evidence-based practice', *British Journal of General Practice*, 52(478): 395–400.

Griffith, R. and Tengnah, C. (2010) *Law and Professional Issues in Nursing: Transforming Nursing Practice*, 2nd edn, Exeter: Learning Matters.

Gurbutt, R. (2006) *Nurses' Clinical Decision Making*, Oxford: Radcliffe.

Nursing and Midwifery Council (2008) *The Code: Standards of Conduct, Performance and Ethics for Nurses and Midwives*, London: NMC.

Nursing and Midwifery Council (2010) *Standards for Pre-Registration Nursing Education*, London: NMC.

Nursing and Midwifery Council (2011) *The Prep Handbook*, London: NMC.

Parahoo, K. (2006) *Nursing Research: Principles, Process and Issues*, 2nd edn, Basingstoke: Palgrave Macmillan.

Pothier, D., Montteiro, P., Mooktiar, M., and Shaw, A. (2005) 'Pilot study to show the loss of important data in nursing handover', *British Journal of Nursing*, 14(20): 1090–3.

Joesph-Williams, N. J., Edwards, A., and Elwyn, G. (2010) 'The importance and complexity of regret in the measurement of "good" decisions: a systematic review and a content analysis of existing assessment instruments', *Health Expectations*, 14(1): 59–63.

Further Reading

Currie, J. (2002) 'Improving the efficiency of patient handover', *Emergency Nurse*, 10(3): 24–8.

Pothier, D., Montteiro, P., Mooktiar, M., and Shaw, A. (2005) 'Pilot study to show the loss of important data in nursing handover', *British Journal of Nursing*, 14(20): 1090–3.

Useful Links and Resources

<http://www.leadershipacademy.nhs.uk/>

The NHS Leadership Academy states that it is part of the NHS and works for all those involved in the health care system: 'We know excellent leadership has a direct, positive impact on our staff and their patients. Our aim is to deliver outstanding leadership, at all levels and across all health professions.' The Academy features several resources relating to clinical decision-making.

8

Leadership, management, team working, and decision making

Mike Lappin

The aims of this chapter are to:

- ➔ enable you to understand the key aspects of both leadership and management in decision making;

- ➔ explore the various theories and models of leadership as they apply to decision making;

- ➔ discuss strategies for managing change, dealing with delegation, and how to motivate individuals and teams; and

- ➔ use real-life case studies from practice as a platform for further discussion of decision making in relation to leadership, management and team working.

Introduction

> *Some of the most influential leaders in an organization don't have a management title. They are leaders because they see what needs to be done, they're willing to take the initiative, and they're able to influence others to work with them.*
>
> (Tye 2009: 137)

It is important that we differentiate between leadership and management right at the outset, and this differentiation can be seen in this statement. However, initially, we will consider both individually and as different facets of what you as a student nurse are required to learn to achieve your competencies to practise as a registered nurse. The concept of team working is explicit throughout this chapter.

Nursing leadership

Recent years have seen the issue of nursing leadership become an important issue for the future of nursing generally, and, most importantly, specifically in relation to the major changes in health and social care, and subsequently in direct nursing care. Patients now require more intensive interventions; bedside technology continues to thrive and, with a more rapid discharge system and quicker throughput of patients in hospitals, many organizations are in search of a workforce who can manage their workload effectively, whilst providing leadership to others.

Employers are looking for qualified nurses who can provide supervision, management, development, administration, and coordination of services to patients and employees (Mahoney 2001: 269). In his letter to the Prime Minister summarizing the interim report of the National Health Service (NHS) Next Stage Review (Department of Health 2007: 3), Lord Darzi set out his aim to convince and inspire everyone working in the NHS to embrace and lead change. Every time you go on duty with an aim to care for patients, whatever their number, you require some degree of skill and potential to lead others to help you to collaborate with your colleagues.

....

⊕ Exercise

Access the interim report authored by Lord Darzi (Department of Health 2007), using the link that appears at the end of this chapter.

What do you notice about what is said about the need for good leadership? How do you think nurses can contribute towards providing the kind of leadership that Darzi advocates?

Access also the final report (Department of Health 2008), again using the link that appears at the end of this chapter, and consider the final recommendations made to enable nurses and other health care professionals to become leaders and managers of care.

Discuss with your tutors how your curriculum is helping you to achieve the required skills and knowledge about which Lord Darzi talks in these reports.

....

The Nursing and Midwifery Council (NMC) *Standards for Pre-Registration Nursing Education* (NMC 2010) now make it explicit how student nurses are expected to achieve competencies in these areas and state in the Standards:

> **Domain 4: Leadership, management and team working**
> **Generic standard for competence**
> *All nurses must be professionally accountable and use clinical governance processes to maintain and improve nursing practice and standards of healt hcare. They must be able to respond autonomously and confidently to planned and uncertain*
> *(Continued)*

> *situations, managing themselves and others effectively. They must create and maxi-*
> *mize opportunities to improve services. They must also demonstrate the potential*
> *to develop further management and leadership skills during their period of precep-*
> *torship and beyond.*
>
> (NMC 2010: 18)

Each field of practice also has its own field-specific competencies related to this domain—that is, competencies that are specific to the main service users that are the focus of the respective field of care.

 Exercise

Consider the field-specific competencies set out in **Box 8.1** in relation to your own field of practice and set yourself a goal during your final placement for achieving these.

Box 8.1 Field-specific competencies relating to Domain 4: Leadership, management and team working

Competencies for entry to the register: Adult nursing

6.1 *Adult nurses must be able to provide leadership in managing adult nursing care, understand and coordinate interprofessional care when needed, and liaise with specialist teams. They must be adaptable and flexible, and able to take the lead in responding to the needs of people of all ages in a variety of circumstances, including situations where immediate or urgent care is needed. They must recognize their leadership role in disaster management, major incidents and public health emergencies, and respond appropriately according to their levels of competence.*

(NMC 2010: 20)

Competencies for entry to the register: Mental health nursing

6.1 *Mental health nurses must contribute to the management of mental health care envi-ronments by giving priority to actions that enhance people's safety, psychological security and therapeutic outcomes, and by ensuring effective communication, positive risk man-agement and continuity of care across service boundaries.*

(NMC 2010: 30)

(Continued)

> ### Box 8.1 (Continued)
>
> **Competencies for entry to the register: Learning disabilities nursing**
>
> 6.1 *Learning disabilities nurses* must use leadership, influencing and decision-making skills to engage effectively with a range of agencies and professionals. They must also be able, when needed, to represent the health needs and protect the rights of people with learning disabilities and challenge negative stereotypes.
>
> (NMC 2010: 39)
>
> **Competencies for entry to the register: Children's nursing**
>
> 6.1 *Children's nurses* must use effective clinical decision-making skills when managing complex and unpredictable situations, especially where the views of children or young people and their parents and carers differ. They must recognize when to seek extra help or advice to manage the situation safely.
>
> (NMC 2010: 48)

Weir-Hughes (2011: 12) declares that it is a myth that only established nurses need leadership skills; he believes that students and newly qualified nurses need them too.

You should also learn to be competent in delegation, have good time management skills, and be able to prioritize your workload and those of others. Keighley (2011: 63) points out that the challenge of developing nurse leadership has been with us since Florence Nightingale raised the issue more than a century ago. The reforms indicated in the Health and Social Care Act 2012 appear to highlight the need for a different framework of leadership from that to which we have been used over the past ten or twenty years and, most importantly from a nurse's point of view, it is now recognized that leadership is required at all levels of the organization.

> ## Activity
>
> Access the Department of Health's series of fact sheets outlining the key themes of the Health and Social Care Act 2012 (see the link at the end of the chapter), and consider the role that nursing leadership might play in contributing to achieving the elements contained within the Act.

In Victorian England, Florence Nightingale had a major influence on the early development of leadership skills and especially in relation to her students, requiring them to focus on total patient care, often reading the 'reflections' of their patient care that they had to record in their notebooks. The overall nursing management of patients was equally as important as the delivery of care.

Mary Seacole's connection to nursing is equal to that of Florence Nightingale, but she also had to overcome racial bigotry and prejudice to become a well-respected figure in nursing. There is now an award named after her that is given for development of leadership (the 'Mary Seacole Leadership Award').

Even by today's standards, both women would be regarded as extraordinary, revealing their own vision of leadership and acting as the premier role models of their time, whilst inspiring their nurses and probationers (student nurses).

For more on Florence Nightingale and Mary Seacole, see the websites listed at the end of this chapter.

Activity

Think about the nurses that have inspired you. What is it about their personal characteristics that makes them inspirational? How might you be seen as a role model by others (fellow students and health professionals)?

Read Thyer, G. L. (2003) 'Dare to be different: transformational leadership may hold the key to reducing the nursing shortage', *Journal of Nursing Management*, 11(2): 73–9, on different kinds of leadership from the more traditional models that you have read about. Make notes of the key issues that the author describes and consider whether the nurses who inspired you were 'transformational leaders'.

Neither leadership nor management sit in a vacuum, however, when considering why they are an important part of your learning to become a qualified nurse. They are also essential to ensuring that quality care is delivered, as well as to engaging with patients and service users to become involved in their own care.

The quality agenda and patient empowerment

We often hear and read about 'quality care', and, as health care professionals, we are concerned with the quality of the service that we provide. Moullin (2003: 5) states that 'it is this which motivates people day in day out in their everyday work which is, in many cases lower paid and more demanding than that of other people in other jobs'. He also highlights that quality:

- is important for patients and service users;
- is important for staff; and
- can help to reduce costs and help us to provide an even better service within a given budget.

Like many student nurses and qualified nurses, you will have chosen a career in health and social care with an aspiration and dedication to caring for the most vulnerable of people, often forgoing a job that may offer you a bigger financial return or a more suitable work pattern.

To make this situation more acceptable, staff need an organized model of work to help them to deliver a quality service. The more disorganized the service, the more demotivated and discouraged they will become. This is where a good leader comes in: a highly motivated leader conveys the vigour and integrity necessary to an excellent organization. Casey and McNamara (2011: 61), for example, point out that 'clinical leadership in nursing and midwifery is particularly important because of the demands of ensuring quality, safety and effectiveness of patient care and inspiring others to achieve likewise'.

Because of your closeness to the patient, this places you in a pivotal position; it demands an appropriate degree of leadership competence, by means of which you must demonstrate the ability to maintain effective care in the face of the ever-present demands on the resources around you.

....

 Exercise

Consider how the ward manager or duty manager in your placement area manages to or-ganize his or her own work and that of others. If possible, negotiate with your mentor and the manager concerned to 'shadow' them for a day, following their daily work. Discuss with them how they see their roles as manager and leader of the staff in their ward, unit, or community field.

Talk then to the nurse in charge about how he or she organizes or prioritizes his or her workload and that of others. How does he or she keep the team well motivated?

Start to formulate plans as to how you might organize your own workload and those of others once you are qualified. What factors might you need to take into account?

....

Bellman (2003) highlights the characteristics of a good leader as including being able to motivate and inspire people. She believes that good leaders are effective commu-nicators, while Freshwater et al. (2009: 124) also point to the fact that nurses have been considered traditionally to be advocates for their patients, meaning that patient empowerment is a key issue. To be an effective advocate, one must also be an effect-ive communicator.

In turn, a good nursing leader will actively participate in this process and work towards a true partnership with the service user. Stanley (2008: 22), however, sees 'the leader as being connected to a process of attending to the needs of their followers so that the interaction of each raises the motivation and energy of the other'. Whilst his paper examines clinical leadership and its relationship to leading staff, it will be clear that such skills are transferable when dealing with the patient population.

Exercise

Consider how nurses act as advocates for patients and for colleagues. How do the nurses use their communication skills to engage in what might potentially be 'difficult' conversations?

Case study 8.1 focuses on a student nurse involved in a situation in practice in which communication, care and delegation are all highlighted.

Case study 8.1 Communication with colleagues, delegation, and prioritizing care

While working on an acute medical ward, I was dealing with a patient who was acutely unwell, with breathlessness and chest pain. Another patient (who had mobility problems) asked me for a commode. I quickly decided that my priority was to the breathless patient. Aware of the need to delegate, I asked a health care assistant (HCA) to bring a commode for the other patient. Once the acute episode was over and my patient was settled, I found out that the HCA hadn't carried out my request, leaving the second patient in some discomfort; he was also fearful of being incontinent as a result.

I was extremely angry that the HCA had completely ignored my request; a member of staff later told me that she dismissed my request, calling me a 'lazy student'!

Question

What action might you have taken if you were the student nurse?

Issues to consider

Sadly, this is an episode from practice that may arise. It is a situation (significant event) in which writing down your experience (reflective summary) may help you to explore your thoughts and feelings about the circumstances involving all aspects of your decision making at the time, including the management of the care of two patients.

It may be that you did not make it clear enough to the HCA that your priority was with the breathless patient, who was at the time acutely unwell, and that this was the reason why you needed someone to help you with the other patient, who had asked for the commode.

Think about the HCA's perception of the situation: he or she may have perceived, because of the way in which you asked her to perform this care task for the patient

(Continued)

Case study 8.1 (Continued)

instead of you, that you simply did not want to do it. If the explanation was not placed in context with the unwell patient, this may have seemed even more of an order rather than a request for help in a difficult decision-making situation.

It would have helped to speak to your mentor about this soon after the event to help you to gain some perspective and a sense of the situation from the HCA's point of view.

This may be difficult for you, but an appropriate action would also be to speak to the HCA in a professional manner to discuss the issues. This will give you an opportunity to hear his or her side of what happened in his or her own words, rather than as reported back to you by someone else. Let the HCA know what you have been told he or she said and explain how that made you feel. It is also important to discuss how the patient whose care needs were not immediately fulfilled must have felt.

Clinical leadership and management

Mahoney (2001: 269) highlighted that 'for nurses to have a voice in the future of health care they need to develop leadership skills and assume leadership positions'. Whether, when qualified, you find yourself a staff nurse providing care for one individual patient or a nurse executive in charge of multidisciplinary departments, in both situations you will need effective leadership skills. As a nurse working within a clinical environment, you will experience many situations in which you will lead both patients and staff alike. Indeed, as a student, you may already be acting in this capacity for some of your peers.

Stanley (2008: 22) conducted a considerable review of the literature, looking for a definitive definition of 'leadership'. His work led him to the conclusion that it is 'seen in terms of unifying people around values and then constructing the social world for others around those values and helping people to get through change'. Bishop (2009a: 6) stated that 'it is important to remember that leadership is needed at every level of health care, particularly at the clinical level where nursing really counts'.

The work of Stanley (2009: 153) supports this. He indicates that junior registered nurses and sisters are the people most likely to be viewed as clinical leaders by their colleagues. Student nurses too have a part to play: you may, for example, have found yourself in a position in which your leadership and management skills are required; your experience and almost constant exposure to such situations will help you to develop the key competencies necessary.

Exercise

Write down some situations in which you have been expected to exercise leadership and management skills.

● Use one of the reflective frameworks from **Chapter 4** to write about one of the situations.

● Think carefully about how you handled the situation and consider alternative courses of action. What alternative actions would or would not work in similar situations and why might this be the case?

Bishop (2009b: 63) highlights that 'leadership in the clinical environment is often derived from the leader's inherent wisdom, personal knowledge, expertise and reputation. While these qualities may be inherited, or perhaps initiated by taking charge in a crisis, they can be learned'.

The good news is that you can learn these skills and continue to grow as a professional, thus enhancing your patient outcomes and adding to the quality agenda. It would appear that a good nursing leader makes clinical excellence possible and Scott (2011: 1) maintains this idea by saying: 'It is simple: it is the quality of nursing that determines the quality of care. That is why nurses should be given much greater freedom and power to take control of what is happening on their wards.'

Mahoney (2001: 270) believes that 'leadership involves learning a body of knowledge, developing skills and, like anything else, lots of practice'. What you need to remember is that the leader's role is not only for those with what may on the surface appear to be some kind of inherent aptitude for leading and who may have what some people call 'charisma', or 'something about them', that makes people follow or take notice of what they have to say. You can, with time, learn the skills of leadership that are required for your first role as a staff nurse and later in your career, as you develop additional knowledge and skills in practice. (See **Chapter 13** for more on making decisions and future continuing education issues after qualifying, and goals for the preceptorship period.)

Marquis and Huston (2012: 31) point out that:

> the relationship between leadership and management continues to prompt some debate, although there is clearly a need for both ... leadership is viewed by some as one of management's many functions; others maintain that leadership requires more complex skills than management and that management is only one role of leadership.

Moullin (2003: 126), however, points to one particularly useful distinction: *management* 'is predominantly activity-based', and is concerned with matters such as planning, budgeting, organizing, and problem solving; *leadership*, on the other hand, involves dealing with people rather than things, creating a sense of direction, communicating the vision, and energizing, inspiring, and motivating. Unlike management, however, Stanley (2006b: 31) notes that 'leadership is not related to seniority in an organization'. The overall aim of leadership is to inspire groups of people to work together to achieve a common goal (Warren 2005). McKimm and Held (2009: 4) highlight that the key message around management and leadership is that successful organizations and teams need both sets of skills and roles, and that neither is superior to the other.

As we have seen, Lord Darzi (Department of Health 2007) was aware of the importance of nurses leading at the point of care and transforming their place of work. On the basis of this report, the NHS Institute for Innovation and Improvement (2009) provided nurses with a planned framework to help them to deliver a higher-quality service while releasing more time to care. The Productive Series published by the Institute (see the link at the end of the chapter) has led to staff engagement, because it empowers them to drive improvements. If you have ever been in a placement in which some members of staff have been a participant in the programme, you will know that the philosophy of this initiative is to permit staff to ask challenging questions about current practices and to make positive changes to the way in which they work.

Case study 8.2 Good leadership: an empowered ward sister

Eileen is a ward sister with a proven track record of leading the quality agenda in all areas of her work. She has a clear vision and excellent communication skills, and her energy and enthusiasm is infectious. She has allowed her staff to add to the process, and has maintained motivation and empowered her team by means of valuing their contribution. She continues to show that she values the group and individuals within that group.

Eileen has been asked to move to a 'failing ward' in order to turn things around. The ward has got a reputation for poor standards of care, staff disengagement, high levels of sickness and absence, and, for some time now, a barrage of complaints with regard to patient care.

Following an initial ward meeting, each member of staff is delegated a project specific to the clinical area: for example, a junior staff nurse is given the task of maintaining an ongoing record of staff development, mandatory training, and appraisals. Another member of staff is given the responsibility of updating, training, and educating staff with regard to the use of infusion pumps and other medical devices in use on the ward.

Weekly meetings are arranged to discuss issues related to the quality of care and improvement agenda. Within a few weeks, the staff in the ward are beginning to embrace this added responsibility and accountability, and there is a feeling that they

(Continued)

Case study 8.2 (Continued)

are now being valued: Eileen is showing them respect and vice versa. This, in turn, increases motivation; staff are now using short- and long-term goals to help them to achieve key performance outcomes.

Staff morale is now high and, within a six-month period, patient complaints have dropped to zero and there had been no reported sickness or absence. Staff begin to approach Eileen with ideas for change, are more productive, and are actively seeking solutions to problems and issues at ward level.

To an outsider, it is quite obvious that the staff are now action-oriented, looking for opportunities to enhance their practice for the benefit of their patients, which has had a positive impact on staff morale and has given them a sense of pride associated with working in such a dynamic environment.

Questions

1. Identify Eileen's style of leadership.
2. What skills and knowledge do you think she has that you will need to develop in leadership and management activities?

You can see from **Case study 8.2** how good leadership can work in practice. Stanley (2006a: 2) argues that 'transformational leaders are described as being connected to a process of attending to the needs of the followers so that the interaction of each raises the motivation and energy of the other'. For Eileen, it was about challenging the ineffectiveness and bringing her vision to the table, sharing that vision, and allowing the staff to take ownership of the situation. Her aim was to get the best out of people, to guide them, teach them, and foster a team approach, whilst at the same time maintaining open communication channels.

Congruent leadership

As a result of his research, Stanley (2006a: 480) proposed the development of a new theory of 'congruent leadership', in which it is not only the way in which someone leads that is important, but also the fact that there is a match between how he or she leads and his or her values and beliefs about what it is that he or she is leading. Eileen, in **Case study 8.2**, showed her leadership approach to be matched by her beliefs about what good nursing care and practice should be on the ward that she had been asked to support.

Consider this issue as you read Stanley's definition of his new theory:

> *The Congruent leader may have a vision and idea about where they want to go, but this is not why they are followed. Congruent Leadership is based on the leader's values, beliefs and principles and is about where the leader stands, not where they are going. Congruent leaders are motivational, inspirational, organized, effective communicators and build relationships. Many have no formal, recognized or hierarchical leadership position and as such Congruent Leadership may offer a better theoretical framework to explain how and why clinical leaders function. Congruent leaders are guided by their passion for care. They build enduring relationships with others, stand the test of their principles and they are more concerned with empowering others, than with power or their own prestige.*
>
> (Stanley 2006a: 480)

 Exercise

You may be taking on some of the leadership functions highlighted in the literature yourself. People may come to ask your advice, or other students may ask you to help them with some nursing interventions or techniques.

- What is it about you and your personal qualities that will make people come to you for this kind of help or advice?
- Do you think that you are someone in whom others believe?
- Are you someone who is 'guided by your passion for care'?
- Is there someone who you think would make a good role model for you to talk to in practice or even in the university?

Reflect on this idea and consider how this quality will be able to help you in your future career choices.

The search for good role models can be never-ending. Many experienced practitioners display a series of rich talents, including a common-sense approach, good listening skills, high levels of academic knowledge, openness and honesty, and also fairness when difficult decisions might have to be made. This will all be demonstrated in a non-calculated way, free from arrogance, and it is this characteristic that will attract 'followers' and gain staff support. It will become clear that this type of leader shows a passion for nursing, treating all people—staff, relatives, and patients—as if they were close colleagues and individuals.

Leadership and the student nurse

To secure the future of the nursing profession, we are going to require good leaders; the revised NMC Standards (NMC 2010) and the accompanying all-graduate profession is the beginning of this challenge. For many of you reading this book, you are part of this future and, as such, learning about decision making in all of its aspects will be essential whatever the field of practice in which you will be working when qualified.

From a leadership perspective, you will have to maintain high standards of care by working together with individuals and teams, respecting them while at the same time upholding the name of the profession. The NMC (2011: 18–19) has highlighted that 'the majority of complaints we receive relate to neglect of care, failure to maintain adequate records, lack of competence and failure to collaborate with colleagues'. All of these factors have a clear link to leadership, management, and team work. As part of this 'securing the future' the Royal College of Nursing (RCN), in collaboration with patient and service organizations, the Department of Health, and the NMC, has developed a key document entitled *The Principles of Nursing Practice* (RCN 2010).

Dr Peter Carter, RCN Chief Executive and General Secretary, explains the purpose of the document as explaining what everyone can expect from nursing and outlining their leadership role in making this a reality:

> *The Principles of Nursing Practice allow us to do just that: they make clear exactly what quality nursing care looks like and provide a framework for supporting the evaluation of care through the development of useful measures. The RCN is committed to driving forward quality improvements—these Principles are an invaluable contribution to that task.*
>
> (RCN 2010)

There are eight guiding principles (Principles A–H), covering such areas as patient dignity, the management of risk, communication, and the importance of team work.

....

 Exercise

Access RCN Principles (RCN 2010) and look, in particular, at Principle H, which includes reference to leadership:

> *Nurses and nursing staff lead by example, develop themselves and other staff, and influence the way care is given in a manner that is open and responds to individual needs.*

Read McKenzie, C. and Manley, K. (2011) 'Leadership and responsive care: Principle of Nursing Practice H', *Nursing Standard*, 25(35): 35–7, an article in a series on the RCN Principles of Practice.

....

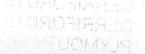

You may have considered some of the knowledge and skills that McKenzie and Manley (2011) discuss earlier in **Part 1** of this book. In the context of leadership, McKenzie and Manley (2011: 35) state that 'leaders should demonstrate good decision making, *problem solving* and *critical thinking* skills' (emphasis added), and in another of the *Nursing Standard* articles on the RCN Principles, Manley et al. (2011: 35–7) note that 'leadership involves *listening*, *interpreting* and confirming understanding, as well as *evaluating* and *reflecting* on the *effectiveness* of the interaction' (emphasis added).

Conclusion

As we have seen in this chapter, both leadership and management skills are required to be an effective qualified nurse who has to work with individual patients and service users, their carers, and their families, as well as with their colleagues in the multidisciplinary team (MDT). Nursing is also about care and you, as a student nurse learning to develop a wide range of skills and knowledge to be able to deliver that care, have to find a way of balancing the decision making that accompanies being a good leader and manager with being a good nurse. This will be challenging for you at times as you make that transition to being an accountable professional practitioner in your chosen field of practice. In **Part 4** of the book, you will see examples of these challenges, and how both leadership and management skills are often indivisible from each other in either managing change at the nurse–patient level or in the wider context of nursing practice as a whole.

References

Bellman, L. (2003) *Nurse-Led Change and Development in Clinical Practice*, London: Whurr.

Bennett, C., Perry, J., and Lapworth, T. (2010) 'Leadership skills for nurses working in the criminal justice system', *Nursing Standard*, 24(40): 35–40.

Bishop, V. (ed.) (2009a) *Leadership for Nursing and Allied Health Care Professions*, Maidenhead: Open University Press.

Bishop, V. (2009b) 'Leaders of the future', *Nursing Standard*, 24(10): 62–3.

Bowles, A. and Bowles, N. B. (2000) 'A comparative study of transformational leadership in nursing development units and conventional clinical settings', *Journal of Nursing Management*, 8(2): 69–76.

Casey, M. and McNamara, M. (2011) 'Learning to lead', *Nursing Standard*, 26(9): 61.

Dawes, D. and Handscomb, A. (2005) *A Literature Review on Team Leadership*, Manchester: The European Nursing Leadership Foundation.

Dean, E. (2011) 'Launch of degree-based curricula marks historic moment for nursing', *Nursing Standard*, 25(51): 12–13.

Department of Health (1999) *Making a Difference*, London: HMSO.

Department of Health (2000) *The NHS Plan: A Plan for Investment, a Plan for Reform*, London: HMSO.

Department of Health (2006) *Our Health, Our Care, Our Say: Making it Happen*, London: HMSO.

Department of Health (2007) *Our NHS, Our Future NHS: NHS Next Stage Review Interim Report*, London: HMSO.

Department of Health (2008) *High Quality Care for All: NHS Next Stage Review Final Report*, London: HMSO.

Department of Health (2011) *NHS Leadership Framework: A Summary*, Coventry: NHS Institute for Innovation and Improvement, University of Warwick.

Freshwater, D., Graham, I., and Esterhuizen, P. (2009) 'Educating leaders for global health care', in V. Bishop (ed.) *Leadership for Nursing and Allied Health Care Professions*, Maidenhead: Open University Press, pp. 121–42.

Hurst, K. (2012) 'Higher staffing levels reduce falls rate', *Nursing Standard*, 26(28): 18–19.

Keighley, T. (2011) 'Leading staff on many fronts', *Nursing Standard*, 25(43): 63.

Kotter, J. P. (1996) *Leading Change*, Boston, MA: Harvard Business Press.

Lewin, K. (1951) *Field Theory in Social Science*, New York: Harper & Row.

Mahoney, J. (2001) 'Leadership skills for the 21st century', *Journal of Nursing Management*, 9: 269–71.

Manley, K. (2000) 'Organisational culture and consultant nurse outcomes, Part 2: nurse outcomes', *Nursing Standard*, 14(37): 34–9.

Manley, K., Hills, V., and Marriot, S. (2011) 'Person-centred care: Principle of Nursing Practice D', *Nursing Standard*, 25(31): 35–7.

Marquis, B. L. and Huston, C. J. (2012) *Leadership Roles and Management Functions in Nursing*, 7th edn, Philadelphia, PA: Lippincott, Williams & Wilkins.

McKenzie, C. and Manley, K. (2011) 'Leadership and responsive care: Principle of Nursing Practice H', *Nursing Standard*, 25(35): 35–7.

McKimm, J. and Held, S. (2009) 'The emergence of leadership theory: from the twentieth to the twenty-first century', in J. McKimm and K. Phillips (eds) *Leadership and Management in Integrated Services*, Exeter: Learning Matters, pp. 20–34.

Moullin, M. (2003) *Delivering Excellence in Health and Social Care*, Maidenhead: Open University Press.

National Health Service Institute for Innovation and Improvement (2009) *The Productive Ward: Releasing Time to Care*, available online at <http://www.institute.nhs.uk/quality_and_value/productivity_series/productive_ward.html>

Nursing and Midwifery Council (2007) *Introduction of Essential Skills Clusters for Pre-Registration Nursing Programmes*, NMC Circular 07/2007 London: NMC, available online at <http://www.nmc-uk.org/Documents/Circulars/2007circulars/NMCcircular07_2007.pdf>

Nursing and Midwifery Council (2008) *The Code: Standards of Conduct, Performance and Ethics for Nurses and Midwives*, London: NMC.

Nursing and Midwifery Council (2010) *Standards for Pre-Registration Nursing Education*, London: NMC.

Nursing and Midwifery Council (2011) *Update: Safeguarding Adults*, London: NMC, available online at <http://www.nmc-uk.org/Documents/Publications-NMC-Update/nmcUpdateMarch2011.pdf>

Ricketts, J. C. and Rudd, R. D. (2002) 'A comprehensive leadership education model to train, teach, and develop leadership in youth', *Journal of Career & Technical Education*, 19(1): 7–17.

Royal College of Nursing (2010) *The Principles of Nursing Practice*, available online at <http://www.rcn.org.uk/development/practice/principles/the_principles>

Scott, G. (2011) 'Mr Cameron must deliver', *Nursing Standard*, 25(37): 1.

Snow, T. (2012) 'Leadership is more important than staffing levels, says Lansley', *Nursing Standard*, 26(28): 7.

Stanley, D. (2006a) 'In command of care: clinical leadership explored', *Journal of Research in Nursing*, 11(1): 20–39.

Stanley, D. (2006b) 'Role conflict: leaders and managers', *Nursing Management*, 13(5): 31–7.

Stanley, D. (2008) 'Congruent leadership: values in action', *Journal of Nursing Management*, 16(5): 519–24.

Stanley, D. (2009) 'Clinical leadership and the theory of congruent leadership', in V. Bishop (ed.) *Leadership for Nursing and Allied Health Care Professions*, Maidenhead: Open University Press, pp. 143–63.

Thyer, G. L. (2003) 'Dare to be different: transformational leadership may hold the key to reducing the nursing shortage', *Journal of Nursing Management*, 11(2): 73–9.

Tye, J. (2009) *The Florence Prescription: From Accountability to Ownership—The Next Frontier for Patient Satisfaction, Workplace Productivity and Employee Loyalty*, Solon, IA: Values Coach, Inc., e-book available online at <http://theflorencechallenge.com/>

Warren, R. (2005) 'What's the difference between managing and leading?', *Christian Post*, 17 October, available online at <http://www.christianpost.com/news/what-s-the-difference-betwe en-managing-and-leading-13770/>

Waters, A. (2012) 'Strategic thinking', *Nursing Standard*, 26(28): 16–19.

Weir-Hughes, D. (2011) 'My guide to clinical leadership: be yourself, listen and engage', *Nursing Standard*, 25(38): 12–13.

Further Reading

Anionuw, E. (2012) 'Mary Seacole: nursing care in many lands', *British Journal of Healthcare Assistants*, 6(5): 244–8.

Bolden, R. (2004) *What is Leadership? Leadership report South West Research Report 1*, Exeter: University of Exeter Centre for Leadership Studies, available online at <https://eric.exeter.ac.uk/repository/bitstream/handle/10036/17493/what_is_leadership.pdf?sequence=1>

Holland, K., Jenkins, J., Soloman, J. and Whittam, S. (Eds.). Second Edition. *Applying the Roper-Logan-Tierney model in practice*, Second Edition. Edinburgh: Blackwell Science.

Useful Links and Resources

<http://healthandcare.dh.gov.uk/act-factsheets/>

A series of fact sheets prepared by the Department of Health to explain the key themes of the Health and Social Care Act 2012.

<http://www.dh.gov.uk/prod_consum_dh/groups/dh_digitalassets/@dh/@en/documents/digitalasset/dh_079087.pdf>

The Darzi Report (interim) (Department of Health 2007).

<http://www.dh.gov.uk/prod_consum_dh/groups/dh_digitalassets/@dh/@en/documents/digitalasset/dh_085828.pdf>

The Darzi Report (final) (Department of Health 2008).

<http://www.florence-nightingale-foundation.org.uk/>

The Florence Nightingale Foundation, which awards scholarships to promote excellence in nursing practice.

<http://www.institute.nhs.uk/quality_and_value/productivity_series/the_productive_series.html>

The NHS Institute for Innovation and Improvement's Productive Series.

<http://www.maryseacole.com/>

A website offering information about Mary Seacole and including a link to the Mary Seacole Centre for Nursing Practice.

<http://www.nursingleadership.org.uk/>

The website of the (European) Foundation of Nursing Leadership.

<http://www.nursingleadership.org.uk/publications/teamreport.pdf>

Dawes and Handscomb (2005) is a review of the literature on team leadership.

<http://www.nursingleadership.org.uk/resources_free.php>

The (European) Foundation of Nursing Leadership offers many free tools and other resources, including a test to identify your leadership style and another that looks at how you work in a team.

<http://www.nwacademytools.org.uk/email/issue_one/pdf/NHS_Leadership_Framework.pdf>

A link to a report on, and reproducing, the NHS Leadership Framework.

Decision making in specific fields of practice

PART 3

This part of the book will focus specifically on the four fields of practice in which student nurses will be undertaking their practice learning and exercising the decision-making skills required to register as a qualified nurse. Each of the chapters is written by a lecturer with experience and expertise in a specific field of practice, and a practitioner who has recently qualified as a nurse in one of the fields of practice. In this way, we hope to ensure that the chapters give examples of recent experiences of decision making in action, linking theoretical concepts with their application and use in the type of real-world experience that student nurses will be expected to manage when qualified. It is intended initially to offer focused decision-making skills to those undertaking each practice pathway and to support the attainment of the field-specific competencies. In keeping with the philosophy of the revised Nursing and Midwifery Council (NMC) Standards (2010), however, the chapters are also of value to students in the other fields of practice, in that an understanding of decision-making situations in the field examined here will enable such students to meet 'exposure to other fields' standards and the generic competencies to which they may apply. Student nurses in any placement will also require, in future, this broader understanding of the care of patients, clients, and their families and carers, which could include the need for essential decision-making skills underpinned by a broader knowledge base.

It is important to note that, in these chapters, the case studies may reflect a specific field or speciality area in which the practice authors have experience of decision making. The important focus is their decision-making development and their reflection on the management of situations in which their knowledge and skills have been 'tested'; these focus on their final-placement experiences as student nurses or a variety of experiences as newly qualified nurses.

9

Mental health nursing and decision making

Tony Warne and Gareth Holland

The aims of this chapter are to:

- ➔ explore a number of interrelated issues in the provision of effective mental health care;
- ➔ explore how relationships between nurses, service users, carers, and other members of the mental health care profession are used to provide effective mental health care;
- ➔ explore, through the use of case studies, how decision making is undertaken in mental health nursing practice; and
- ➔ enable student nurses to learn how and why effective decision making is essential to developing and maintaining therapeutic relationships.

Introduction

The chapter first explores the issues involved in how and why mental health nurses come to learn about the decisions that they need to take in clinical practice, and why these are crucial to the establishment and maintenance of therapeutic relationships. It must be noted that various terms will be used throughout this chapter that refer to individuals requiring care and support from nurses—that is, 'patients', 'service users', and 'clients'.

We will also explore some of the challenges and tensions that can arise when there is a difference between what the professional and the service user might feel is the right decision. Reference is made to the prevailing mental health legislation in the United Kingdom and, in particular, the legislation around care being provided possibly against an individual's wishes and while he or she is living in the community. If you are not living or studying in the UK, you should seek out the relevant legislation that applies to your country. You might want to see where the similarities and differences are between that and the UK legislation.

The chapter concludes with a discussion of how the mental health nurse can ensure that inclusive and informed decision making leads to safe, secure, and effective mental health care. By means of the case studies and the discussion, it will enable you, as the student nurse, to learn how different kinds of decision making can influence outcomes of care, and it will also help you to work towards achieving the Nursing and Midwifery Council (NMC) competencies as they relate to decision making in nursing practice.

Note that while the case studies are based on real-life examples of decision-making situations, all names in the case studies have been changed, in keeping with *The Code: Standards of Conduct, Performance and Ethics for Nurses and Midwives* (NMC 2008).

Mental health nurse education, practice, and research

Mental health nurse education, practice, and research have long championed innovative approaches to improving our understanding of the impact, on individuals, the communities in which they live, and wider society, of the decisions and actions taken in the name of therapeutic endeavour. However, improved understanding does not always lead to better decisions being taken by those that have this knowledge.

Many mental health nurses have experienced similar difficulties and challenges in developing their own practice and the teams within which they work. Sometimes, these difficulties have been very complex. For example, like other areas of nursing, in mental health nursing there has long been a theory–practice debate. This debate centres on the argument that the classroom is dominated by theoretical knowledge, with practical knowledge being the domain of clinical practice, with rarely any connection between these two different, but related, knowledge areas (Freshwater and Stickley 2004). For many mental health nurses, however, there has also been an ongoing theory–theory debate, which has challenged the way in which mental health nurses have carried out their practice (Chambers 2006).

Preparing for mental health nursing

While some students might relish these debates and discussions, for other students these debates can be uncomfortable, and they can challenge these students' self-confidence as people and as aspiring professionals (Warne and McAndrew 2010). From an educational perspective, it has been argued (Warne and McAndrew 2007) that contemporary approaches to the educational preparation of mental health nurses require rethinking.

It should be possible to think about concepts of 'preparedness' as being both educational and emotional precepts, so that both the technical and theoretical knowledge required for practice and the attitudes and emotions that influence the individual in practice might be more effectively aligned. It is possible that you will have thought more about this when you have experienced these two aspects not being aligned.

....

 Exercise

Think back to the very first clinical placement on which you went.

- How prepared did you feel for the particular area of practice?
- How did you feel when thinking about starting the first shift?

Take a moment to think back and reflect on these two aspects, and consider what you would have liked to have known about the practice area and how that might have made you feel. If you have not yet undertaken your first placement experience, you can consider what you have been told about that placement or what you have discovered. What are your feelings about how prepared you think you are for that first day?

....

This first exercise should help you to think about a concept of preparedness that acknowledges the interrelated and entangling space between 'knowledge' and 'knowing'. Just as theoretical knowledge is considered implicit in delivering good practice, knowing also forms part of our ability to deal with our interpersonal relationships within the context of our external world. Reeder (2002) has argued that there is a difference between these two concepts:

- *knowledge* is described as a conscious secondary process relating to the information residing in our minds;
- *knowing* is an unconscious primary process that influences the way in which we use knowledge.

Knowing is a product of our upbringing and background, which encompasses our beliefs and values, and is culturally and socially bounded.

....

 Exercise

Consider how knowledge of mental health nursing is required to enable you to make decisions that relate to you personally and also to those concerning patients or service users whom you will meet in practice. In addition, consider whether this knowledge actually helps you, as a person and as a student nurse, to know how to make decisions in practice. Discuss the possible answers with your mentor or personal tutor.

If you are undertaking a mental health nursing placement, but you are following another field-of-practice pathway—for example, adult nursing—are there any differences between this and your knowledge of mental health nursing that will impact on your experience in that placement? Think about how the generic competencies under the NMC *Standards for Pre-Registration Nursing Education* (NMC 2010) can be used in a different field of practice from your own.

In relation to mental health nursing practice, however, it is the mental health nurse's attitude to 'knowledge' and his or her aptitude for 'knowing' that will allow him or her to explore and make sense of his or her own and other people's experiences, feelings, needs, and motives. The ability to 'know me' in order to learn better how to 'understand you' is the crux of the therapeutic relationship, and is central to the notion of providing 'holistic care' (Warne and McAndrew 2010). We will consider this in the context of decision making, but it is essential first that you understand what we mean by a 'therapeutic relationship'.

The therapeutic relationship

The therapeutic relationship is central to effective mental health nursing. Such relationships require the individual nurse to be attentive, to be able to hear the patient's story, and at the same time to provide safety by containing the story and the expressed personal philosophy, or inherent beliefs and values, of both the patient and the nurse.

It has been suggested, however, that for some individuals the processes of self-examination and interpretation necessary to establish and maintain effective therapeutic relationships might be threatening and confusing (Warne and McAndrew 2007). Many nurses, particularly those at the beginning of their professional careers, strive to possess *all* of the knowledge and skill required to be a competent and effective nurse. However, perhaps it is that we *do not yet know* those things that might be important in terms of becoming and being an effective mental health nurse. For example, novice nurses complete their education and training possessing countless skills and much relevant theoretical knowledge. Yet what many of these novice professionals lack is the knowing required to ensure that such knowledge is used in a meaningful way in relation to the unique individuals with whom they will be working. Recognizing this uniqueness reflects another strand of knowledge that might also be useful to consider—that is, patient experience knowledge—and with this the emotionality of the interpersonal space that this knowledge can create between the nurse and patient (see **Figure 9.1**).

Whilst decisional models mostly favour a rationalist view of evidence (Hastie and Dawes 2001), it has been argued that service user experience is a 'third strand' of evidence (Rycroft-Malone 2004). However, whilst acknowledging service user experience and the value of evidence derived from qualitative studies, this is often qualified with the rider that the 'best' evidence is drawn from quantitative methods, with consequent emphasis on standardization techniques.

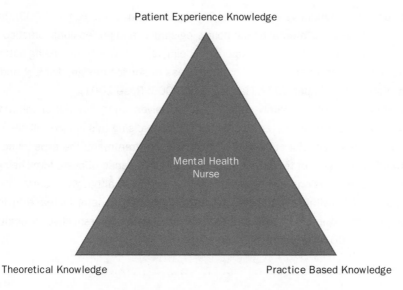

Figure 9.1   The three major sources of knowledge for mental health nurses.

So there can be some resistance to acknowledging and valuing patient experience knowledge, and such resistance can be difficult to overcome. We argue here that, in achieving effective decision making in mental health care, being able to embrace the choices and preferences of service users is something that every nurse needs to try consciously to build into his or her approach to providing care.

⊕ Exercise

Think about a situation that you have experienced in which your mentor discussed with a service user how he or she wanted to be involved in his or her own care. What decisions did the service user make? What knowledge did he or she have to support his or her knowing how to make that decision? Discuss with your mentor how he or she felt in enabling the service user to make decisions about his or her own care.

This major change in mental health nursing practice from making decisions *for* service users (patients) rather than *with* them could be considered a radical one.

Making decisions: partnerships between nurse and patient

In thinking about how to achieve a greater sense of partnership between nurse and patient, the shift required is from decisions based on professional values towards those based on patient values (Fulford 2004; Woodbridge and Fulford 2003). In many international settings, mental health policy, legislative, and professional practice trends have revealed a more determined approach being taken towards increasing patient and public involvement within the democratic process of service design, delivery, and evaluation (Happell and Roper 2002; Happell et al. 2003; Rose 2001).

Many patients will ultimately decide for themselves what they will or will not do in regard to any treatment offered or provided, and exercising this choice will have an impact upon the successful outcomes of any particular treatment, the experience of any untoward side effects of treatment, and an individual's sense of overall well-being. How patients make decisions is not always well understood, although interest in patient decision making within mental health care reflects the general increase in interest in patient-centred interventions that focus on the patient perspective in health care (Lauver et al. 2002; van Dulmen 2003).

....

⊕ Exercise

For a good example of how such a major change in mental health nursing practice (that is, the 'paradigm shift') has occurred, read Warne, T. and McAndrew, S. (2007) 'Passive patient or engaged expert? Using a ptolemaic approach to enhance mental health nurse education and practice', *International Journal of Mental Health Nursing*, 16(4): 224–9.

This is a paper that explores the reason why so many of us, when we become service users, become content for others to make decisions on our behalf. Take some time to think about the last shift during which you were working (and learning) in practice. Can you identify three things that were said or done by nursing colleagues that might unintentionally have disempowered service users?

....

Much has been said in earlier chapters about decision-making theory and how such theories might be applied in health care. Indeed, much has been written about clinical decision making and its relationship with information-processing theory (Newell and Simon 1958) and social judgement theory (Lauver et al. 2002), and until recently much of this work has focused upon medical decision making. Shared decision making represents a radical divergence from the traditional model of the health care professional as a paternalistic authority (Nelson et al. 2001). In mental health care, such approaches usually involve a number of interrelated elements of decision making:

(1) Information

In this context, what we mean by 'information' is all that is required in order to make a particular decision—although what this information consists of can be different depending on who has the information, how it is to be used or prioritized, and who is processing this information when making a decision. For example, the doctor might use information represented by the signs and symptoms observed when deciding on treatment options. If these treatment options include, say, the prescribing of medication, then the likely known efficacy of the particular drug will be noted, the usual prescribing range consulted, and perhaps reactions to other medications being taken might also be considered. While we may know it, we may or may not disclose other information, such as the probabilities of risks, benefits, and lifestyle changes associated with taking a particular medication. In mental health, it is often these considerations that form the basis for decision making around compliance and not the information on therapeutic value, for example (Gask and Rogers 1998; Sirey et al. 2001).

(2) Values

It's clear that different values reflect the importance that people place on information for decision making, as well as on various aspects of their experience and other factors in the broader context of their encounters with mental health care services (Woodbridge and Fulford 2003). In the formal clinical decision-making situation (prescription of medication, for example), quantitative estimates of values are drawn upon that act as proxies for the desired end point of health and well-being, and these are used to balance out any negative aspects of treatments.

For example, depressed patients often place high importance (value) on feeling better, but might also value avoiding adverse treatment side effects. The relative strength of these values can significantly impact patient preferences for treatment options, subsequently affecting the choices that patients make about treatments (Cooper et al. 2000; Gask and Rogers 1998).

(3) Decision-making context

At any one time, it will be the context within which these relative values are explored that will influence an individual's decision making within the broader context of his or her life, and this may sometimes be a powerful influence on the choices that a patient makes. Used here, 'context' refers to the various aspects of an individual's day-to-day life and functioning, as well as the health care system structure and process, and the broader socio-cultural milieu that shapes people's experiences. So, in our example of a service user's being prescribed medication for a mental health problem, as well as information on the therapeutic value and the relative value on quality of life, other considerations might include the perceived social stigma associated both with seeking help and with complying with professional mental health service interventions (Link et al. 2001).

(4) Preferences

As the service user considers these sometimes competing strands of information, it is almost inevitable that, in some circumstances, the decision-making choices will be ranked in order of preference. Preferences represent a relatively greater liking of one alternative as compared to (an)other alternative(s).

Using an extreme example from a non mental health care setting, but an example that is clearly going to impact upon an individual's physical and mental health and well-being, consider the decisions that some patients diagnosed with cancer have to make. For the individual, it might be a choice between surgery, radiotherapy, or accepting no treatment. In mental health, even with the advent of new neuroleptic drugs, there is evidence to suggest that service users often feel that the choice of treatment for those with serious mental illnesses is not really a choice (Bunn et al. 1997).

These four decision-making elements—information, values, decision-making context, and preferences—should be as important for the mental health nurses as they will be for the service user (Happell et al. 2004). Recognition of the importance of these four elements is crucial for developing an approach that sees the mental health professional able and willing to provide information to service users in a way that puts the needs of the service user first (Bridson et al. 2003).

....

⊕ Exercise

1. Consider what a nurse might need to ensure is included in an approach to the assessment and review of long-term medication with service users that promotes the preferences of the service user.
2. What difficulties do you think might be involved for the:
   (a) service user?
   (b) mental health nurse?
   (c) other members of the mental health team?
3. What do you consider to be the differences between patient-centeredness and service-user involvement and participation in shared decision-making processes?

....

Decision making in practice

In many circumstances in which nurses work with colleagues from other disciplines in providing mental health care services, it is often the nurse who will be in a prime position to ensure that shared decision making routinely forms part of the care-giving approach (Welsh and Lyons 2000). It is nurses who usually have the greatest contact with service users. It is this consistency in the provision of care that requires the mental health nurse to develop expert communication and interpersonal relationship skills (Warne and McAndrew 2007).

One area of mental health nursing practice in which this can be seen is in the assessment and monitoring of service users' progress against agreed treatment or care plans to ensure that these remain optimal. As we noted in **Chapter 4**, in these situations it is possible that some mental health nurses might approach such assessments with a well-developed intuitive 'feel' for what might be going on, yet will remain constrained by the limitations imposed by their training and an uncritical acceptance of empirically based evidence.

Indeed, it has long been noted that most health care professionals do not make clinical decisions based simply on intuition (English 1993; Guyatt et al. 2001). However, in many therapeutic situations, in which the mental health nurse's ability to communicate and develop relationships are paramount, a fundamental conflict may arise between the need to respond immediately to service-user needs and the considered systematic processes demanded by 'science'.

Schon (1983), in his famous work on the reflective practitioner, argued that practitioners do not always operate using a technical rational basis, and do not routinely or consciously draw upon all of the separate forms and information available to them every time they are faced with the need to make a decision in clinical practice. Indeed, sometimes other considerations come into play, as **Case study 9.1** illustrates.

Case study 9.1 Decision making as a newly qualified nurse

I can remember when I was working on my first shift as the only qualified member of staff on the ward, approximately a month into my preceptorship period. I was working with two support workers, neither of whom were regular ward staff, but who were experienced colleagues. The ward itself was unsettled when two patients, Paul and Michael began fighting at the end of the bedroom corridor. I had no idea what had caused the fight, but immediately I ran to the situation, pulling my personal alarm for the first time as I did so.

The fight was stopped without any serious injury to either of the patients, but Paul began to make a number of threats to harm himself and Michael if he wasn't immediately moved off the ward.

Paul had a diagnosis of borderline personality disorder (BPD), and a history of prolific and extreme self-harm, and I felt that these threats were potentially genuine. Following a discussion with the senior (and very experienced) nurse who had attended the ward in her role as the duty manager, the decision was made to place Paul on one-to-one observation.

As a result, no further violent incidents took place. However, the following day, I was informed by my ward manager that, according to the unit policy, patients shouldn't be placed on one-to-one observation as a result of a threat of self-harm.

(Continued)

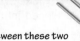

Case study 9.1 (Continued)

While I believe that the decision I made prevented any further violence between these two patients, with hindsight I don't believe that it was the right one.

In the heat of the moment, I relied on the advice of senior nurses, because of my lack of knowledge of the policies of the unit on which I was working and a lack of awareness of what might be considered an appropriate management of someone with a BPD diagnosis.

Of course, at that time, I was also not very confident in my own skills as a newly qualified nurse.

Issues to consider

The nurse in this situation was inexperienced and was facing being in the position of the only qualified nurse on duty at the time. The first decision taken was to deal with the situation before it escalated and he followed the correct procedure. As he ran to the situation, he communicated via his personal alarm that assistance was required. The immediate problem was dealt with and the potentially difficult situation was contained.

However, as the stabilized situation changed, the nurse was faced with having to make decisions that were outside of his knowledge and experience. Again, understanding the need to gain advice, he relied upon the judgement of a very senior and experienced nurse to take the decision to care for one of the service users involved on a one-to-one basis, thus reducing the risk of further harm occurring either to service user or to anyone else.

So far, it would be possible to argue that the 'correct' decisions had been taken. It was only the following morning that an alternative way forward was revealed. Partly, this was described as being 'unit policy', but such a policy would have been developed from an evidence base and best practice experience—which, for this nurse, was at that time unknown. Interestingly, perhaps, when the nurse had a chance to reflect, he thought that he had not taken the right or best decision.

It was clear that, in this case, the nurse was unable to respond to the wider problem, and his decision making was focused on the one or two aspects that could be dealt with using the information and knowledge that he had available to him. Arguably, this is not unusual. Hicks (1998) has noted that, as nurses have increasingly rejected the task-oriented approach to care in favour of a more holistic approach, reliance on empirically based evidence to shape nursing practice has only a limited part to play. She argues that every experienced nurse will be able to recall situations in which they have drawn on their tacit knowledge and experience to respond immediately to the needs of the situation, without necessarily considering whether

(Continued)

Case study 9.1 (Continued)

this might have led to the best decision being taken. The newly qualified nurse's post-decision-making action was to reflect on the situation in order to learn from the whole experience. As seen in **Chapter 4**, this revisiting of the scenario as a whole enabled him to consider the actions of everyone involved, as well as the feedback given by the ward manager.

So it is clear from **Case study 9.1** and its possible outcomes that, for mental health nurses, learning to negotiate appropriate care within complex environments necessitates deep understanding of the process of decision making. Models differ in their theoretical position, but share the same drive towards decisions based on sound reasoning, transparency, and evidence (Woodbridge and Fulford 2003). As can be seen from **Case study 9.1**, for both nurses and service users, there might be inconsistencies in the value placed on different sources of evidence. Variations exist that can create ethical and practice dilemmas for mental health nurses attempting to work in non-coercive, person-centred ways whilst being cognizant of the evidence underpinning care (Rycroft-Malone 2004; Thompson and Dowding 2002).

Case study 9.2 allows us to explore some of these dilemmas.

Case study 9.2 Managing a difficult situation

During my first experience of night duty as a qualified nurse, I worked every shift as the only qualified member of staff on the ward, and I found the patient group extremely challenging. One patient in particular had been involved in a number of incidents. Tom was an 18-year-old male with a history of violent assaults on staff and other patients, a tendency to acquire and use weapons in these assaults, and on a previous admission he had taken another patient hostage. Shortly after the ward bedtime, Tom and another patient had refused to go to bed, preferring to pace around the day area in an attempt to intimidate staff. Despite numerous

(Continued)

Case study 9.2 (Continued)

requests from myself and support workers to go to bed, the two patients refused; at one point, Tom walked to his bedroom and returned almost immediately with his fists clenched. His body language was extremely aggressive and I noticed that he had something sticking out of his fist. I asked him what he had in his hand; he said 'Nothing' and continued to walk towards me in a very intimidating manner. I asked him again and told him to open his fingers, which he did, revealing a very sharp, 3″ screw, which fell out of his hand and under the (locked) door of the kitchen.

With the immediate danger managed, I asked Tom to sit and talk with me in an attempt to de-escalate the situation without the need to activate my alarm—which he did. He became noticeably calmer during our conversation (although I can't remember what we talked about) and eventually retired to bed, and I felt happy with the decision that I had made because no one had been injured or harmed in any way.

However, during the handover in the morning, my colleagues on the early shift were appalled that I had neither pulled my alarm nor placed Tom in seclusion. I was made to feel as though I'd placed everyone I work with in extreme danger as a result of this decision, which was confirmed when, later that day, unable to sleep I phoned the ward to speak with my manager who confirmed that I should have activated my alarm *and* secluded Tom, and that the nursing team on the early shift had taken the decision to seclude Tom as a precaution whilst they reassessed the risk that he posed to staff and patients.

I had made the decision partly on an instinctive reliance on my communication and emerging nursing skills, and partly because I believe that, had I pulled my alarm and a response team attended the ward, this would have caused a much more dangerous situation in that Tom would have felt threatened or challenged, and would have been likely to react with violence. However, once the immediate danger had been dealt with, I believe that I should have attempted to manage the long-term risks that Tom posed by determining whether he had further weapons or had genuinely intended to cause someone harm.

Approximately two months later, we received information from another patient that Tom had acquired a metal pen, which he was hiding in his bedroom and sharpening in order to 'stab up' a member of staff. In light of the feedback regarding my earlier decision in managing Tom, I arranged to have his bedroom searched and, upon finding said pen and because of Tom's inability to deny that he would harm someone with it, I and the other qualified nurse on shift made the decision to seclude Tom to manage his pronounced risk to others. (The decision this time was a shared one, taken with another colleague and also influenced by the previous experience of needing to check a decision that I considered the right one to take.)

However, following this decision we were informed by the manager that this was not a decision that we should have made, because it was not entirely in line with our policies regarding the use of seclusion and the risk was not sufficient to justify it. Making decisions in practice are complex, but in each of these situations the main issue was the prevention of risk of self-harm and harm to others that was the outcome in both situations.

What **Case study 9.2** brings to light is the argument that the stages of the decision-making process can be deconstructed and that, in doing so, decision-making behaviour can be improved (Thompson and Dowding 2002). Whilst there is general agreement that a decision involves a retrievable store of organized knowledge arising from prior experience, with consequent options and choices, when used in the context of mental health nursing, much of the literature emphasizes professionals' options and choices—their using of their 'expertise'—rather than collaborating with the end user. In **Case study 9.2**, such collaboration was not possible, but a solution presented itself on which the nurse decided rather than risk taking a different, but possibly an expected, response.

Whilst mental health nurses should be making 'good' decisions based on sound and reliable evidence, what constitutes 'good' in mental health practice often remains subject to the preferences of the various professional stakeholders involved in an individual's care and treatment. Likewise, it has been noted that relying on the available 'best evidence' can have limited utility for the ambiguity of decision making when applied to individualized, person-centred approaches to care (Faulkner and Thomas 2002). However, Rolfe (2005a, 2005b, 2006) argues that such practice ambiguity can be addressed by clinically active staff using reflection as the vehicle for producing contextualized evidence.

Person-centeredness shifts health care away from an exclusive focus on symptoms and physiological outcomes, because service users often value functional outcomes and their quality of life more highly than they value control of the illness (Noble and Douglas 2004). So, in shared decision making, the mental health nurse strives to become a consultant to the service user, helping to provide information, to discuss options, to clarify values and preferences, and to support the service user's autonomy.

Case study 9.3 Becoming more experienced

Whilst working a night shift, I was asked to provide cover for another acute ward that had no qualified nurse available at the beginning of the shift. Although I'd finished my preceptorship a couple of months before, suddenly being placed on another ward forces you to try to establish rapport with new individuals. It is something that any nurse should be prepared for when qualified.

One of the patients on the ward, Carl, had been diagnosed as having no treatable mental illness and was awaiting a transfer back to prison. Carl was a young man with a history of violence, drug abuse, and prolific self-harm when faced with stress. Also, Carl had been

(Continued)

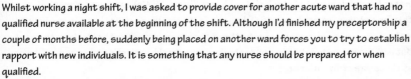

Case study 9.3 (Continued)

involved in tattooing himself and other patients on the ward, which posed a significant risk of infection and some safeguarding issues. Staff had been unable to ascertain how he was doing this, and were faced with hostility and occasionally violence whenever they attempted to intervene. Carl's argument was that, because he had no mental illness, then how could staff in a hospital justifiably restrict his actions. He used the act of tattooing himself as a coping strategy, albeit a poor one, in order to avoid acts of deliberate self-harm.

On this particular night, I spent a long time engaging with Carl during one-to-one sessions, because he was experiencing stress as a result of arguing with his girlfriend on the phone and I felt that I had established the foundation of rapport with him. He remained awake throughout the night and, at around 4 a.m., he was found by staff doing routine checks to be tattooing his forearm in his bedroom. I approached Carl and spent some time talking with him in his bedroom. He was using a safety pin, which he had acquired from some clothing brought in for another patient, and he had used a contraband lighter to sterilize it. He appeared quite agitated and said that he would assault any member of staff who attempted to prevent him from tattooing himself, and that he would also seriously self-harm if restrictions were put in place to prevent him from acting as he chose.

I returned to the nursing office to discuss the issue with the staff with whom I was working, who were unsure and looked to me to make a decision as nurse in charge. I weighed up the situation and decided to take a course of action that I believed would resolve the issue without causing unnecessary distress to the patient and without causing risk to staff. I spoke with Carl again and told him that I would allow him to finish tattooing his arm only if he agreed that, when he had finished doing so, he handed in the safety pin and allowed me to clean the site. He agreed, and a short time later approached me and happily complied with my requests.

This decision was a complex one, because I had to consider a number of factors. What would have been my reasons for intervening, had I chosen to do so? This patient had been diagnosed as illness-free and would undoubtedly have deliberately harmed himself significantly, and potentially my colleagues, if we had attempted to restrain him. I believe that it would have caused him great distress to be restrained, particularly when his actions were affecting only himself and he had not posed a risk to others. I was also viewing it in terms of 'safe self-harm', in that he was already at high risk of blood-borne viruses (BBVs) as a result of previous tattoos and years of intravenous (IV) drug use. In allowing me to clean the wound and handing in the pin, Carl allowed me to manage further risk, thereby increasing the safety of the ward. But perhaps most importantly, I made the decision with the patient's wishes and well-being at the centre of my rationale.

At times since qualification as a nurse, these two factors have often appeared to be mutually exclusive, and very hard to reconcile. I'd have been entirely justified (not to mention

(Continued)

Case study 9.3 (Continued)

covered by policy) if I'd chosen to restrain Carl, to strip his room of further items that could be used to self-harm, and then to manage a volatile, angry, and potentially violent man accordingly.

However, I wanted to see him as a person, one who was perfectly capable of deciding what to do with his own body and deserved the opportunity to make these choices. I was worried that I could have been accused of being 'soft' by colleagues, of giving a challenging patient exactly what he wanted in order to avoid conflict, but I'd never wanted to create difficult situations simply based on policy. While they are necessary and at times protective, policies can sometimes provide shelter for bad decisions, or even a lack of decision making, while confidence, experience, and instinct are often far more reliable and flexible. So much nursing education teaches (or attempts to teach) mental health nurses to consider each patient as an individual and I tried to do so here. Rather than managing the situation by forcing Carl to act in the manner that I felt was appropriate, I managed the person, thus allowing him to manage the situation himself, to maintain his dignity and (relative) freedom, and to live his life.

Issues to consider

What this situation illustrates is that decision making in clinical practice often relies upon an approach that is sometimes described as being intuitive, drawing upon prior expertise (Benner 1984). It has been argued that adopting such an approach can lead to poor decision making that results in unsatisfactory outcomes for all concerned (Thompson and Dowding 2002).

The case study illustrates that perhaps not all decisions can easily be found in the textbooks. This nurse was faced with someone who, on the face of it, had a legitimate claim to be left alone to do what he wanted to do, albeit there were possibly some personal risks involved. There are several issues that have become entangled in this case. The patient was awaiting transport back to prison, because it had been decided he did not have a mental illness that might have contributed to his criminal behaviour. Although there can be a connection between mental illness and criminal behaviour, this is not always the case. Out of 1,564 people convicted for homicide in England and Wales between April 1996 and April 1999, only 164 (that is, 10 per cent) were found to have had symptoms of mental health problems at the time of the offence (Department of Health 2001). This is a proportion that remained fairly constant over the next ten years.

Given this figure, and the between fifty and seventy cases of homicide a year involving people known to have a mental health problem at the time of the murder,

(Continued)

Case study 9.3 (Continued)

there is insufficient evidence to support the sensationalized media coverage about the danger that people with mental health problems present to the community (Large et al. 2008).

However, when this patient had been challenged previously by ward staff about his behaviour, the patient had often responded with hostility and sometimes violence. The member of staff had limited resources available to him and a number of other patients on the ward to keep safe.

The patient was a long-term illicit drug user and had self-tattooed before, and on this occasion he was using an implement that could not be considered sterile, thus increasing the risk to his own health and well-being, and possibly that of others around him.

Finally, the nurse in charge was also aware of the ward policy on how to deal with potentially disruptive and violent behaviour, and he was also aware that other colleagues might challenge the decisions that he took on the basis that non-conformity with norms might make it difficult for others to make decisions in the future.

As the nurse observed, the case was a complex one.

⊕ Exercise

1. Consider what you might have done in the above situation. What ethical issues do you think might arise from looking after someone in a mental health service who does not have a recognizable diagnosis?

2. Which concern do you think was the most important one to take into account when making a decision: the personal safety of the patient and staff; the right to behave in the way in which the patient wanted to; or ensuring that the health of the patient was not compromised by the amateur tattooing?

3. Should limited resources ever be part of a professional decision-making process? If so, to what ethical dilemmas might this give rise?

In **Case study 9.3**, the nurse drew upon a number of interpersonal factors in his decision making. These appear to have been kindness, genuineness, civility, and respect. Effective nurse–patient communication is at the heart of shared decision making.

Effective communication will enable, as in this case, the patient's perspective and contextual factors that might impact upon the quality of the interaction with the nurse to be taken into account (Roter 2003).

However, arguably, being an effective communicator requires something beyond developing and utilizing an effective interpersonal style. It also requires the nurse to harness the insight available from the way in which his or her beliefs and assumptions developed from previous experiences influence the judgements and choices that he or she makes within the decision-making process of care delivery.

The key to effective involvement in decision making is the relationship established between the patient and the mental health nurse. These are likely to be relationships that are supportive, and which reinforce the feeling of being heard and a sense of being valued as equals. Whilst **Case study 9.3** illustrates that the relationship does not have to be explicitly therapeutic to also be effective within mental health care, patients do not find it helpful to be told what to do or think, or to have their actions judged. What is valued is help and support that can strengthen their pre-existing coping strategies, and which recognizes their expertise (Warne and McAndrew 2007).

Adams and Drake (2006) have argued that, in therapeutic practice, the most helpful decisions are those that strengthen existing coping strategies rather than those that weaken them. Achieving effective nurse–patient participation in shared decision making will also facilitate decisions taken to be transparent and open to scrutiny. While such an approach will benefit the patient, such transparency will also help a nurse to deal with anxieties such as those expressed by the nurse in **Case study 9.3** regarding the judgements that his colleagues might make about the decisions he took in resolving the particular decision.

Conforming to organizational norms has been the subject of much work, from the famous psychological studies carried out by American psychologist Milgram (1963) to more contemporary studies that have looked at why people conform to organizational norms (for example, see Smith et al. 2007). For the newly qualified and appointed mental health nurse, there is great ontological security to be gained in conforming. In so doing, the individual avoids harm and stress by means of the protection of the group. Equally, however, the group can be oppressive and harmful to those who do not conform (Warne and McAndrew 2007).

We do not know how, in **Case study 9.3**, the nurse's colleagues responded. We can see, however, from reading the reflection, that they looked to the qualified nurse recounting the experience as the 'nurse in charge' to make the final decision. But it is to be hoped that his explanation for pursuing a shared approach to decision making and, in this example, for achieving a positive outcome would have been a persuasive one, and the nurse's decision would have been accepted as the best one to have taken in that set of circumstances.

Conclusion

A greater emphasis has been placed on involving patients in the decisions taken over their treatment and care. Collaborative or shared decision making in professional practice reflect a shift in focus from professional values toward the values of service users. Patients can be experts as a result of their experiences and their experience of their mental health problem must be seen as unique, whatever understanding there may be about a particular diagnosis or condition. The challenge for mental health nurses is to develop and nurture the organizational and professional norms that embrace and harness the values of patient participation at the level of individual care and decision making.

References

Adams, J. and Drake, R. (2006) 'Shared Decision making and evidence base care', *Community Mental Health Journal*, 42(1): 87–105.

Benner, P. (1984) *From Novice to Expert: Excellence and Power in Clinical Nursing Practice*, Menlo Park, CA: Addison Wesley.

Bion, W. R. (1963) *Elements of Psycho-Analysis*, London: Heinemann.

Bridson, J., Hammond, C., Leach, A., and Chester, M. (2003) 'Making consent patient centred', *British Medical Journal*, 327(15): 1159–61.

Bunn, M., O'Connor, A., Tansey, M., Jones, B., and Stinson, L. (1997) 'Characteristics of clients with schizophrenia who express certainty or uncertainty about continuing treatment with depot neuroleptic medication', *Archives of Psychiatric Nursing*, 11(5): 238–48.

Chambers, M. (2006) 'The case for mental health nurses', in J. Cutcliffe and M. F. Ward (eds) *Key Debates in Psychiatric/Mental Health Nursing*, London: Churchill Livingstone, pp. 33–45.

Cooper, L., Brown, C., Vu, H., Palenchar, D., Gonzales, J., and Ford, D. (2000) 'Primary care patients' opinions regarding the importance of various aspects of care for depression', *General Hospital Psychiatry*, 22(3): 163–73.

Department of Health (2001) 'Safety First', *Report of the National Confidential Inquiry (NCI) Into Suicide and Homicide by People with Mental Illness* – Annual report: England and Wales. Department of Health.

English, I. (1993) 'Intuition as a function of the expert nurse: a critique of Benner's novice to expert model', *Journal of Advanced Nursing*, 18(3): 387–93.

Faulkner, A. and Thomas, P. (2002) 'User-led research and evidence based medicine', *British Journal of Psychiatry*, 180: 1–3.

Freshwater, D. and Stickley, T. (2004) 'The heart of art: emotional intelligence in nurse education', *Nursing Inquiry*, 11(2): 91–8.

Fulford, K. (2004) 'Ten principles of values-based medicine', in J. Radden (ed.) *The Philosophy of Psychiatry: A Companion*, New York: Oxford University Press, pp. 205–34.

Gask, L. and Rogers, A. (1998) 'Bridging the gap: mapping a new generation of primary mental health care research', *Journal of Mental Health*, 7(6): 539–41.

Guyatt, G., Haynes, B., and Jaseschke, R. (2001) 'The philosophy of evidence-based medicine', in G. Guyatt and D. Rennie (eds) *User's Guide to the Medical Literature: Essentials of Evidence Based Clinical Practice*, Chicago, IL: American Medical Association, pp. 403–9.

Happell, B. and Roper, C. (2002) 'Promoting consumer participation though the implementation of a consumer academic position', *Nurse Education in Practice*, 2(2): 73–9.

Happell, B., Manias, E., and Roper, C. (2004) 'Wanting to be heard: mental health consumers' experiences of information about medication', *International Journal of Mental Health Nursing*, 13(4): 242–8.

Happell, B., Pinikahana, J., and Roper, C. (2003) 'Changing attitudes: the role of a consumer academic in the education of postgraduate psychiatric nursing students', *Archives of Psychiatric Nursing*, 17(2): 67–76.

Hastie, R. and Dawes, R. (2001) *Rational Choice in an Uncertain World: The Psychology of Judgement and Decision Making*, Thousand Oaks, CA: Sage.

Hicks, C. (1998) 'Barriers to evidence-based care in nursing: historical legacies and conflicting cultures', *Health Services Management Research*, 11(3): 137–47.

Hopton, J. (1996) 'Reconceptualizing the theory–practice gap in mental health nursing', *Nurse Education Today*, 16(3): 222–32.

Kuhn, T. (1970) *The Structure of Scientific Revolutions*, 2nd edn, Chicago, IL: University of Chicago Press.

Large, M., Smith, G., Swinson, N., Shaw, J., and Nielssen, O. (2008), 'Homicide due to mental disorder in England and Wales over 50 years', *The British Journal of Psychiatry*, 193: 130–3.

Lauver, D., Ward, S., Heidrich, S., Keller, M., Bowers, B., and Brennan, P. (2002) 'Patient-centred interventions', *Research in Nursing & Health*, 25(4): 246–55.

Link, B., Struening, E., Neese-Todd, S., Asmussen, S., and Phelan, J. (2001) 'The consequences of stigma for the self-esteem of people with mental illness', *Psychiatric Services*, 52(12): 1621–6.

Milgram, S. (1963) 'Behavioural study of obedience', *Journal of Abnormal and Social Psychology*, 67(4): 371–8.

Nelson, G., Lord, J., and Ochocka, J. (2001) *Shifting the Paradigm in Community Mental Health: Towards Empowerment and Community*, Buffalo, NY: University of Toronto Press.

Newell, A. and Simon, H. (1958) 'Elements of a theory of human problem solving', *Psychological Review*, 65(3): 151–66.

Noble, L. and Douglas, B. (2004) 'What users and relatives want from mental health', *Current Opinion in Psychiatry*, 17(4): 289–96.

Nursing and Midwifery Council (2008) *The Code: Standards of Conduct, Performance and Ethics for Nurses and Midwives*, London: NMC.

Nursing and Midwifery Council (2010) *Standards for Pre-Registration Nursing Education*, London: NMC.

Reeder, J. (2002) 'From knowledge to competence: reflections on theoretical work', *International Journal of Psychoanalysis*, 83(4): 799–809.

Rose, D. (2001) *Users' Voices*, London: The Sainsbury Centre for Mental Health.

Rolfe, G. (2005a) 'Validity, trustworthiness and rigour: quality and the idea of qualitative research', *Journal of Advanced Nursing*, 53(3): 304–10.

Rolfe, G. (2005b) 'The deconstructing angel: nursing, reflection and evidence-based practice', *Nursing Inquiry*, 12(2): 78–86.

Rolfe, G. (2006) 'Judgements without rules: towards a postmodern ironist concept of research validity', *Nursing Inquiry*, 13(1): 7–15.

Roter, D. L. (2003) 'Observations on methodological and measurement challenges in the assessment of communication during medical exchanges', *Patient Education and Counselling*, 50(1): 17–21.

Rycroft-Malone, J. (2004) 'Research implementation: evidence, context and facilitation— the PARIHS framework', in B. McCormack, K. Manley, and R. Garbett (eds) *Practice Development in Nursing*, Oxford: Blackwell, pp. 118–47.

Schon, D. (1983) *The Reflective Practitioner: How Professionals Think in Action*, San Francisco, CA: Jossey Bass.

Sirey, J., Brue, M., Alexopoulos, G., Perlick, D., Friedman, S., and Meyers, B. (2001) 'Perceived stigma and patient-rated severity of illness as predictors of antidepressant drug adherence', *Psychiatric Services*, 52(12): 1615–20.

Smith, J. R., Hogg, M. A., Martin, R., and Terry, D. J. (2007) 'Uncertainty and the influence of group norms in the attitude–behaviour relationship', *British Journal of Social Psychology*, 46(4): 769–92.

Tee, S., Lathlean, J., Herbert, L., Coldham, T., East, B., and Johnson, T. J. (2007) 'User participation in mental health nurse decision making: a cooperative enquiry', *Journal of Advanced Nursing*, 60(2): 135–45.

Thompson, C. and Dowding, D. (2002) *Clinical Decision Making and Judgement in Nursing*, London: Churchill Livingstone.

van Dulmen, S. (2003) 'Patient-centeredness', *Patient Education and Counselling*, 51(3): 195–6.

Warne, T. and McAndrew, S. (2007) 'Passive patient or engaged expert? Using a ptolemaic approach to enhance nurse education and practice', *International Journal of Mental Health Nursing*, 16(4): 224–9.

Warne, T. and McAndrew, S. (2010) 'Learning at the edges of knowing and not knowing', in T. Warne and S. McAndrew (eds) *Creative Approaches to Health and Social Care Education*, Basingstoke: Palgrave, pp. 232–9.

Welsh, I. and Lyons, C. (2001) 'Evidence-based care and the case for intuition and tacit knowledge in clinical assessment and decision making in mental health nursing practice: an empirical contribution to the debate', *Journal of Psychiatric and Mental Health Nursing*, 8(4): 299–305.

Wills, C. and Holmes-Rovner, M. (2006) 'Integrating decision making and mental health interventions', *Clinical Psychology*, 13(1): 9–25.

Winnicott, D. (1971) *Playing and Reality*, London: Routledge.

Woodbridge, K. and Fulford, B. (2003) 'Good Practice? Values based practice in mental health', *Mental Health Practice*, 7(2): 30–4.

Further Reading

Tee, S., Lathlean, J., Herbert, L., Coldham, T., East, B., and Johnson, T. J. (2007) 'User participation in mental health nurse decision making: a cooperative enquiry', *Journal of Advanced Nursing*, 60(2): 135–45.

Wrycraft, N. (ed.) (2009) *An Introduction to Mental Health Nursing*, Maidenhead: Open University Press.

Useful Links and Resources

<http://standards.nmc-uk.org/PublishedDocuments/Standards%20for%20 pre-registration%20nursing%20education%2016082010.pdf>

Pages 22–30 of the NMC Standards (2010) cover competencies for mental health nursing.

<http://www.mentalhealth.org.uk/>

The Mental Health Foundation website links to many publications and resources, including a literature review on mental health capacity and Mental Health Capacity Act 2005, which is focused on decision making with individuals in a variety of situations in which this Act is relevant.

<http://www.samhsa.gov/>

The US Substance Abuse and Mental Health Services Administration (SAMSAH) website includes numerous resources that support shared decision making with service users. While these are set in the context of a US health care system, the key concepts are transferable to that of the UK.

10

Decision making in children's and young people's nursing practice

Aatefa Lunat and Denise Major

The aims of this chapter are to:

- ➔ consider decision making in the context of children's and young people's nursing;
- ➔ offer examples of decision making in action through reflection and clinical case studies; and
- ➔ consider how decision making can be developed to achieve the competencies required by the Nursing and Midwifery Council.

Introduction

The purpose of this chapter is to address decision making in the field of children's and young people's nursing practice in relation to the field-specific competencies outlined by the Nursing and Midwifery Council (NMC) in the *Standards for Pre-Registration Nursing Education* (NMC 2010). In order to explore these competencies further, we will consider examples from practice, and links will be made between the various examples from practice and the competencies in order to demonstrate their importance. To allow an in-depth exploration of the examples from practice, we will use Johns' (1994) model of reflection. 'Reflection' is described as a means by which nurses can closely examine their theoretical knowledge along with their nursing practice (Johns 2000). The process of reflection has been found to have great benefits for nurses, because it allows them the opportunity to change and develop practice in order to carry out improved care practices (O'Regan and Fawcett 2006). In this chapter, the evidence of decision making has been interlinked with critical evidence-based reflective practice, and demonstrates its integration and development in the role of the newly qualified nurse.

The chapter will begin by discussing examples derived from practice, and key aspects from these examples will be taken and related to the NMC Standards (NMC 2010). The chapter will then go on to discuss key elements required to make decisions in clinical practice. The evidence base for many of the decisions taken in the case study is interwoven throughout the narrative, thus enabling you see how they link together in nursing practice.

Decision making in practice: the newly qualified nurse

Centred on a newly qualified staff nurse on the neonatal unit, the single case study around which this chapter is structured considers the care of a sick neonate whose parents were adolescents. This example was chosen because it illustrates many aspects of caring decisions that have to be made for patients from birth through adolescence, because the parents themselves were still in the later stages of childhood.

The case study itself appears as dialogue, and the Standards and competencies referred to are those generic and field-specific competencies that a student pursuing a children's nursing field-of-practice pathway is required to achieve, found under the heading 'Competencies for entry to the register: Children's nursing' in the NMC Standards (NMC 2010).

Let us begin by hearing from the newly qualified nurse:

> After making observations of the behaviour of the young parents with the baby on several occasions, I noticed that they were holding back from engaging when invited by staff to help to care for their baby. The parents didn't ask any questions and their responses were very limited when they were spoken to by staff, comprising only the one-word answers that Wolfe et al. (2006) suggests are typical of teenagers, owing to their insecurity of knowledge during the psychosocial stage of Kohlberg (1969).

Cole and Cole (2001) describe how, at the age of 15, young people's social worlds revolve around the closeness of their friends and the positive self-esteem that joining in with friendship activities gives them.

It was obvious that the parents were comfortable with each other's company, because they talked freely to each other when staff weren't in the close vicinity—but they didn't talk to the staff and assumed an air of not being able to join in with the caring for their baby. The parents weren't observed spontaneously picking the baby up nor did they ask if they could do so or how to pick up their baby; hence they had very little physical contact with their baby for the first seven or eight days of her life. The young parents had very limited skills and knowledge about the care of a baby, and had difficulty bonding with their baby. They often said that they felt that they were unable to ask questions and to communicate their views, because they lacked confidence.

I felt that I had to intervene, to help them to bond with the baby, so as to increase their chances of developing a positive parenting relationship, which would increase their family relationship in later times and support the child's physical, social, and psychological development (Bee and Boyd 2007).

Competency 1.1 of 'Domain 3: Nursing practice and decision making' (NMC 2010: 44) requires that children's nurses must be able effectively to recognize the needs of people who come into their care and must be able to respond to their needs by taking appropriate action.

Clinical decisions and clinical judgements are important elements of nursing practice, because they have a direct effect on patient care (Clack 2009), so I spoke to senior staff on the unit and told them about the concerns I had about the parents' lack of input to the care of their baby.

Competency 1 of Domain 3 highlights that decisions made in partnership with staff involved in the care of the patient will ensure that high-quality care is provided (NMC 2010: 44). By discussing concerns with senior members of staff and informing them of what she planned to do next, staff were able to clarify that what the newly qualified nurse was planning to do could have a positive effect on the parents. Competency 4.1 of 'Domain 1: Professional values' (NMC 2010: 41) requires that children's nurses must be able to work in partnership with young people and their families using a family-centred care approach, to plan and deliver the required support and care. This is further supported in Competency 4 of Domain 3 (NMC 2010: 45), which states that the physical, social, and psychological needs of people must be met throughout different life stages to enable better quality of life. Therefore while these young people were not actually patients themselves, they had developed needs of their own in terms of learning how to care for their baby as they approached adulthood.

> Because I was working a number of consecutive shifts on the unit, I was able to build up a rapport with the parents and an effective therapeutic relationship. I spent time in encouraging them to get involved in caring for their baby, by asking them if they wanted to change their baby at care times, to prepare feeds, to hold the baby, and to feed the baby. I reassured the parents by telling them that I would help them and would be available to advise them whenever needed.

According to Competency 6 of 'Domain 2: Communication and interpersonal skills' (NMC 2010: 43), it is essential that every nurse takes the opportunity to provide education and health promotion through effective communication. The newly qualified nurse employed a framework often used on the neonatal unit to assess how competent the parents were in caring for their baby. The framework comprised a discharge checklist, which incorporated practical skills such as bathing the baby, sterilizing bottles, preparing feeds, and general care of the baby, in which parents are expected to demonstrate competence before their baby is discharged home. The discharge checklist is representative of good practice guidance, as outlined in Gomes (2010) as a measure of supporting inexperienced parents in their parenting skills.

Competencies 5 and 5.1 of Domain 3 (NMC 2010: 45) also state that a wide range of tools must be used to assess young people and their families in order to improve health and well-being by promoting health and social inclusion. Using the framework allowed this newly qualified nurse to identify those areas in which the young parents needed the most support. By spending valuable time with the parents, she helped gradually to increase their confidence in asking questions, and they began to appear to be happier and more content. It is a key requirement of competency 1.1 of Domain 2 (NMC 2010: 42) that the individuality and stage of development of each child must be taken into account in order to involve young people and their families actively in the decision-making process. Here, the developmental stage of the infant required that, as a nurse, the newly qualified nurse ask the parents what they already knew and help them to learn what was needed to enhance their child's development. As a nurse, she felt that this was a good decision, because it enabled her to identify the areas in which the parents required the most support and it also allowed her to work collaboratively with the parents.

> When I initially met the young parents, they were very reserved and lacked confidence. I felt sad to see how they struggled to bond with the baby and also that they didn't feel confident enough to seek support and guidance.

According to the Field standard of competence for Domain 1 (NMC 2010: 40), children's nurses must act as advocates for children, young people, and their families. It is essential that children's nurses work in partnership with families to empower them and to enable them to voice their views, worries, and concerns—but it is also important that the nurse tries not to become too emotionally involved in the matter.

Peplau (1952) states that to be present when a patient and his or her family are going through a difficult situation and not to become enmeshed by it is an attribute of maturity as a nurse. It is important to remember that increased parental anxiety may decrease the amount of involvement to which some parents feel able to commit themselves (Coyne 1995). Warren (2010) further states that, by addressing parental concerns, an atmosphere will be created in which parents will feel more confident about engaging in their baby's care. For communication to be effective, according to Competency 2.1 of Domain 2 (NMC 2010: 42), it is important the children's nurses have a good understanding of child development from infancy to young adulthood, in order to enable young people to gain a better understanding of health care needs and also to enable them to contribute to making decisions.

> After I intervened and offered the parents support, I felt it was very rewarding to see the change in how the parents interacted with their baby.

Competency 8 of Domain 3 (NMC 2010: 46) expresses the importance of providing young people and their families with educational support and self-care skills in order to maximize their knowledge, skills, and abilities to care for themselves, and also to improve their understanding when making decisions.

> As a newly qualified member of staff, I initially was unsure of my views and concerns about the young parents because of my lack of experience in caring for young parents, so I clarified my views with senior members of staff, who also agreed that they were concerned about the parents.

. . . .

⊕ Exercise

Think of a situation in which you have recently been involved that required you to make a decision. Write down three things that concerned you about making the decision.
    Consider why it concerned you.

. . . .

You might have thought about the following issues:

- being unsure about unit policy to support the decision;
- feelings of having to meet colleagues' professional expectations of you;
- making a wrong decision that could jeopardize your registration; and
- not knowing the extent to the boundaries of decision making—that is, how much to do alone and what decisions should be made by more senior staff.

A key recommendation of Competency 6.1 of 'Domain 4: Leadership, management and team working' (NMC 2010: 48) is that children's nurses must effectively use their clinical decision-making skills when managing complex situations. They must also be able to recognize when they may need the support and advice of senior staff to enable safe practice.

> I also felt as though I may have been out of my depth in making decisions such as putting a support plan in place for the young parents. I felt that I lacked confidence in intervening with the young parents, because I was still in the transitional period of student nurse to staff nurse, and still felt that I had limitations to my role as a student would.

Standard 8 of Domain 1 (NMC 2010: 41) also points out that all nurses must be aware of their limitations, and must seek advice and guidance from senior staff if they feel that they lack competence or knowledge in order to provide high-quality care.

....

 Exercise

What potential actions did you consider when making the decision in the first exercise?

....

You might have considered the following.

- Perhaps you discussed the issue with your mentor or preceptor, or your manager?
- Did you read any local or national professional guidelines?

> A similar event to this one had occurred when I was a student in my first year. However, as a student, I merely observed my mentor and was unable to make decisions at the time because of the early stage of nursing education at which I was and also because I did not have enough knowledge to make a sound decision. On this occasion, though, my professional reputation required me to make a sound decision
>
> *(Continued)*

regarding how I could solve the problem presented to me by the parents, and my knowledge and previous experience allowed me to identify that the young parents required health promotional learning (NMC 2008).

The following areas in which I had developed knowledge and experience aided my decision:

- parenting skills in relation to bonding theories;
- child-centred care; and
- teaching in the form of 'parentcraft'.

I was initially unsure of my feelings and observations of the behaviour of the young parents; so I clarified my views with senior members of staff. I learned that, when making decisions as a newly qualified member of staff, I could use different sources such as guidelines, frameworks, and senior members of staff to clarify my decisions. The informal clinical supervision that I was able to seek was another mechanism that supported me in making a decision.

If a similar event were to occur again in the future, I wouldn't be afraid to trust my intuition and feelings, and I'd feel confident in approaching senior staff when I felt as though I needed extra support and guidance.

Benner (1984) describes intuition as a deep understanding of the background of a situation and it is that what makes an expert different from a novice. I'd also feel confident intervening with support for the parents, because I now feel that I've gained great experience in this area. After the event occurred, I felt a change in position in the nursing team.

As a newly qualified staff nurse, I often felt that I lacked confidence in voicing my opinions and concerns. I think that this was because I was afraid that I may be looked upon as incompetent by the senior staff nurses, who were a lot more highly skilled and knowledgeable than I was. I felt, as a result of the event, that I was able to demonstrate my skills to the staff on the unit, and show that I was proficient in making decisions and able to seek support when needed. This demonstrated to them that I was a safe practitioner and enabled me to take a more active role in the team. I now feel like a valued member of the team, and feel as though my opinions and views are appreciated.

A longitudinal study carried out by Spouse (2001) identifies that the way in which pre-registration students and newly qualified staff see themselves as nurses is highly influenced by the way in which their fellow colleagues accept them and welcome them into their team.

After the event, I was able to reflect back on the situation with a senior member of staff, who applauded me for my actions. After the positive feedback that I received, I realized that I'd started to develop in my role as a staff nurse on the neonatal unit and that my self-confidence had grown, enabling me to take a more self-directed approach in my role, because I felt assured that I could ask more senior staff for help and support when needed.

Competency 10 of Domain 3 (NMC 2010: 46) and Competency 4 of Domain 4 (NMC 2010: 47) express that evaluation, supervision, and learning from experience is key to improving clinical decision making and personal development. One of this newly qualified nurse's future learning needs was to gain a better understanding about child development from the perspective of both the neonate and the parents.

We can see here that learning to make decisions is dependent on having the best underpinning knowledge and skills with which to enter into a shared care relationship with parents. For those of you who are undertaking a course of study in the children's nursing field of practice, some understanding of child development will enable you to link the underpinning knowledge required as it applied to both parents and child.

Child development theory

According to Spano (2003), adolescence is a time of physical, cognitive, social, emotional, and interpersonal changes. There are a number of different theories that focus on adolescent development. In this particular event, the parents of the neonate were both adolescents. The mother was 15 years old and the father was 16. According to Piaget's (1972) stages of cognitive development, the parents fall within the 'formal operational' stage. At this stage, adolescents begin to develop the ability to think logically and adopt skills such as deductive reasoning and systemic planning; thus the thoughts of young people at this stage are very similar to those of adults (Cole and Cole 1993).

When the young parents visited their baby on the neonatal unit, they found it difficult to be affectionate towards her. They were often very hesitant to touch their baby when I offered them the opportunity and often displayed feelings of embarrassment, such as by giggling on handling the baby, and their very tense posture when holding the baby showed that they were uncomfortable and were unsure of how to interact with her.

Although the young parents were at the formal operational stage of Piaget's theory in other aspects of life, they were unable to fulfil this stage as parents. It has been outlined by Piaget (1972) that adolescents may not always demonstrate formal operational thoughts when they are unfamiliar with particular tasks. In this case, parenthood was an unfamiliar situation to the young parents.

Activity

Take into account, and make observations of, the behaviours and attitudes that adolescents often display, and consider how decision making can best be managed based on these observations.

Discuss these with your mentor and personal tutor.

Erikson (1956) explored the social and emotional development of children and adolescents. Erikson's theory is broken down into eight stages, which are known as the 'eight stages of man'. Each stage is described by Erikson as a 'psychosocial crisis', which arises and needs to be resolved before the next subsequent stages can be managed as a socially and emotionally healthy individual (Child Development Institute 2011). The adolescent parents fall within the 'identity versus confusion' stage of Erikson's (1956) theory. During this stage, adolescents consider their identities and also what they aspire to become in the future. In an idealistic situation, by the end of this stage, the young adolescent should develop an idea of who they are and what they would like to do in the future (Erikson 1956).

Initially, the young parents experienced great difficulty at this stage. This may have been the result of role confusion, because they had to come to terms with identifying themselves as parents and also because they were unsure of what parenthood would entail. Erikson (1956) claims that identity confusion can make adolescents feel extremely uncomfortable and could, in turn, hinder their chances of accomplishing the stage at which they are. After much encouragement and support was delivered to the adolescent parents, they eventually began to come to terms with their role as parents, and also started to show love and affection towards their baby. They displayed confidence and maturity when taking full responsibility for the care and feeding of their baby, and started to make decisions as parents.

⊖ Top tips

When making decisions in practice:
- Identify the problem in relation to which the decision is being made.
- Consider factors contributing to the problem.

- Think about what actions could reduce or eliminate the contributing factors.
- Consider the support mechanisms that are available in your area of practice for yourself and for the patient.
- Put in place actions that will reduce contributing factors using the support mechanisms that you have identified.

The first stage of Erikson's (1956) theory is 'basic trust versus mistrust', and this stage usually occurs from birth to 1 year old. This stage would have a significant impact on the neonate of the adolescent parents. During this period of life, babies decide if their surrounding environment is safe. When the infant is well handled, nurtured, and loved, he or she will develop a sense of trust and security (Erikson 1956). On the other hand, infants who have not had their basic and emotional needs met may decide that the world in which they live is a hostile one, and therefore they may find it difficult to form relationships in the future owing to their development of insecurities and mistrust (McLeod 2008). Research has shown that the children of adolescent parents may attain less in life than the children of adult parents. It has been suggested that this may be as a result of biological factors such as young parental age and developmental immaturity in young parents (Chen et al. 2007). This demonstrates the impact of bonding and parental involvement on the neonate (Child Development Institute 2011), and also the importance of support and encouragement by nursing staff, as stated in Competency 8 of Domain 3 (NMC 2010: 44).

> Prior to the baby's discharge home, the adolescent parents frequently came to visit their baby, and tended to all of her feeds and care throughout the day. They were able to work together to care for their baby and showed that they were able to meet her physical, emotional, psychological, intellectual, and social needs. This demonstrated that they took full parental responsibility for their baby and had a good understanding of what parenthood entailed. The adolescent parents also displayed a stronger, more mature and loving relationship between themselves. I was amazed to see how the parents first came to the unit as young adolescents and how they developed into young adults.

The behaviour that the adolescent parents displayed prior to their baby's discharge home showed that they had quickly moved on to Erikson's (1956) next developmental stage, which is 'intimacy versus isolation'. During this stage, young adults consider whether they would like to live alone or settle down with a partner. Although this stage is usually completed at a later stage of life, in this situation the adolescents, as parents, were able to initiate the stage by becoming a strong parental unit with a constructive relationship between them.

Mental health foundation: young people and resilience

Good mental health allows children and young people to develop the resilience to cope with whatever life throws at them and to grow into well-rounded, healthy adults (Mental Health Foundation 2011). Resilience occurs when children do well despite the risk factors in their lives. Risk factors are stressors that have proven or presumed effects in increasing the likelihood of maladjustment in children (Gutman et al. 2010).

The Department of Health (2006) states that the main risk factors contributing to adolescent pregnancy include poverty, children in care, children of adolescent mothers, low educational attainment, not being in education, sexual abuse, mental health problems, crime, violence, and bullying. The risk factors for the stressors of resilience and teenage pregnancy have many similarities between them, and therefore may have contributed to the adolescents in question becoming adolescent parents.

There are many protective factors contributing to adolescent resilience that have been outlined by the Mental Health Foundation (2011). They include the adolescent's need to feel loved and valued, to live an optimistic and enjoyable life, to be able to learn and succeed, to accept who he or she is and to recognize what he or she is good at, to have a sense of belonging in his or her family and community, to be able to feel that he or she has some control over his or her own life, and to have the strength to cope when something is wrong and to develop the ability to solve problems (Mental Health Foundation 2011).

Poor emotional health not only affects the well-being of the young parents, but also affects their ability to be attentive and nurturing parents, which can lead to an increased risk of accidents and behavioural difficulties for their child. Some young parents may have pre-existing poor emotional health, but this is exacerbated by the demands of parenthood, particularly when they lack family support, are in conflict with each other, or are isolated in poor-quality housing (Department for Education and Skills 2006).

Evidence (Department for Education and Skills 2006) shows that strong social and emotional skills help to shape young people's levels of self-awareness and self-esteem, their ability to build relationships and to empathize with others, and their levels of motivation and confidence in taking control of their lives. Therefore early identification and appropriate support for adolescent mothers and fathers with poor mental and emotional health is needed in order to allow improved outcomes both for the adolescent parents and their children (Health Development Agency 2007).

As a registered nurse, recognizing signs of emotional stress in parents may be the first step towards deciding how to include them in their child's care.

....

 Exercise

Consider what behaviours in parents might cause you to be concerned about their ability to engage in care or would make you concerned about the child's safety if they were included in care. It is a good idea at this point to write down your ideas and to identify areas about which you need more knowledge to make an initial decision on the types of behaviour that would cause you concern and on which you would have to make decisions.

....

Ethical principles

In neonatal care, decisions are often made on behalf of babies by their parents or, in some cases, by health professionals in the context of surrogate decision making as a result of the non-autonomous state of the newborn baby (Spence 2000). 'Autonomy' refers to the respect that should be shown for an individual's ability for self-determination and his or her own personal goals (Wyatt 2010). In the case of pre-autonomous individuals, respect can be shown by ensuring that parents are given the responsibility to consent to treatment on behalf of their baby (Glasper and Richardson 2006). It is important to remember that, as nurses, we have a primary responsibility to communicate as fully as possible with parents and to involve them in all aspects of their baby's care (Spence 2000). It is vital that parents are involved in all decisions relating to their infant on the neonatal unit, especially prior to their baby's discharge home. Cagean and Meier (1983) point out that parents often experience less anxiety when they know that they will be included in the discharge planning process.

Activity

Take time out to have a conversation with parents on your next placement and to find out in what aspects of care they would like to be involved in relation to their child. Is there any difference between the issues in which one set of parents would like to be involved and those of another? Why do you think there might be differences?

Top tips

Communicating with parents in the form of negotiated partnership may allow you to:

- identify parental anxieties;
- identify aspects of care with which the parents may wish to be involved; and
- adapt nursing care to help parents to get involved with their baby to the level that suits them.

⊕ **Exercise**

Consider occasions within the ward environment on which it may not be beneficial for the parents to deliver care to their infant or child.

You may have thought of the following occasions:

- a child/infant who has been newly ventilated;
- an unstable or critically ill child/infant;
- a child/infant who is receiving post-operative care, who may be at risk of wound dehiscence or increased pain; or
- a child/infant who may be at risk of displacing an arterial line, drain, etc.

Surrogate decision making in neonates differs from all other forms of decision making, because it entails making a decision on the behalf of a neonate who is non-autonomous and therefore has not yet developed interests (Beauchamp and Childress 1983). When making decisions, it is important to act in beneficence rather than non-malificence. 'Beneficence' refers to the duty of providing benefit and 'non-malificence' refers to the duty of not inflicting harm (Wyatt 2010). In the case of a neonate, relevant interests would include comfort, well-being, and future development (Spence 2000). It has always been a value of neonatology that every baby deserves the best medical treatment and care that can be provided, and also that every effort should be made to protect him or her from harm or abuse (Wyatt 2010).

> *Occasions often occurred on which the adolescent parents had to consent to treatment or plans of interventions, such as newborn hearing screening and screening for retinopathy for their baby.*

It is vital to remember that parents have a central role in participating in all treatment decisions, and that staff must develop an open, respectful, and collaborative relationship with the parents from the beginning in order for the best decision to be reached (Wyatt 2010). In these situations, it was important that the parents fully understood what they were consenting to or that they had the right to refuse consent. It has been suggested that the way in which adolescents interpret words often differs from how they will interpret them when they are adults and can lead to miscommunication (Biehl and Halpern-Felsher 2001). Therefore it is vital that nurses and other health professionals do not assume that adolescents have fully understood the message conveyed, because this can significantly affect the decision-making process. Gormley-Fleming and Campbell (2011) also state that if parents are not fully informed of the treatment to which they are consenting, they will find it difficult to reach an informed decision.

According to the Department of Health (2001), if the mother of a child is under 16 years of age herself, she will be able to give valid consent for her child's treatment only if she is deemed to be *Gillick* competent in order to make the decision required (so-called after the case that gave rise to the rule). In this case, it would be lawful for the decision to be made on the basis that it is in the child's best interest (Department of Health 2001). In this specific situation, the parents had a good understanding of the interventions to which they were consenting and they were competent in making such decisions.

According to Wyatt (2010), it is essential that all staff caring for neonates understand the fundamental ethical and legal principles that encircle their nursing practices. Nurses involved in neonatal care have the duty always to act in the baby's best interests. The principle of always acting in the baby's best interest is particularly important when caring for neonates, owing to their unique vulnerability and dependence on others for all aspects of their care (Wyatt 2010).

Neonatal care should be provided with the belief that every baby, however small or sick, has value as would a healthy individual. The United Nations Convention on the Rights of the Child, which entered into force in 1990, states that children everywhere have the right to life, the right to survival and development, the right to protection from harmful influences, abuse, and exploitation, and the right to participate fully in family, cultural, and social life. Wyatt (2010) states that it is both a legal and moral requirement that every baby is in possession of these rights from birth.

Advocacy is also a key concept used in neonatal care, because it is based on the fact that there will always be someone who will need someone else to speak out on his or her behalf to protect his or her best interest (Glasper and Richardson 2006). Neonates who have not yet achieved the developmental skills for autonomous decision making are a prime example of this (Mallik 1997).

> There were several occasions on which the young parents felt intimidated by doctors and other senior staff. This made them feel uncomfortable in approaching the medical staff with any questions or concerns, and also hindered their own decision making abilities. I often acted as the advocate for the young parents and their baby by conveying their expressed thoughts to the medical staff.

The newly qualified nurse's advocacy role is evident in the way in which she worked with the young parents to gain their consent to a treatment regime. Negotiation with the child and family has been found to have enabled a more positive approach, with everyone acting in the child's best interests (Huband and Trigg 2003). Thus it was paramount that the nurse made a positive decision to embrace the responsibility of advocacy, in order to promote inclusivity of the parents so as to empower them in their baby's care, and thus promote a stronger family bond for future social unity and strong emotional health.

Transition from student to staff nurse: professional growth

> During my first few weeks of working on the neonatal unit, I felt as though I spent a great deal of time trying to get to know my colleagues and showing them how competent I was in my role as a staff nurse. I felt as though I was spending a lot of my time making sure that everything was done on time, because I was conscious that I was taking a lot longer to complete tasks in comparison to my colleagues and I didn't want them to think that I lacked in time management and organizational skills. I was afraid that this may affect how I was accepted as part of the team.
>
> I sometimes felt intimidated when working with senior staff on the unit, because I felt that they had such high expectations of me and, as a result, I felt I had to perform my new role at the level expected by them without revealing to them how difficult I was actually finding the transition in to my new role. Duchscher's (2008) 'transition shock' model identifies this as the physical response to the transition experience. The changes through which I went as part of my transition were stressful and exhausting.

Exercise

Consider actions that you might take to gain acceptance when commencing a placement in a new clinical area.

 Top tips

The type of preparations that you make as a student can also help you in your new role as a staff nurse, because they communicate your learning needs to your new supervisor, preceptor, or buddy.

- Be prepared—undertake a self-assessment against the role requirements and prepare personal professional development plans that identify your learning needs.
- Identify who your allocated supervisor, preceptor, or buddy is.
- Introduce yourself and give a little background of your previous experiences.
- Speak up regarding your own cognitive or experiential level.
- Share your plans with your supervisor, preceptor, or buddy.
- Gain stability in one area of care before accepting a more difficult challenge.

(Duchscher 2007; Major 2010)

I found it very hard to be responsible in making clinical judgements and practice decisions, because I always felt doubtful as a result of my lack of experience. This resulted in a lack of confidence and insecurity. Higgins et al. (2009) state that the increase in responsibility and accountability has been found to bring with it increased stress, tension, anxiety, and pressure. This has been broken down further by Clark and Holmes (2007) into a number of areas, which include management and organizational skills, prioritizing care needs, time management, delegation, drug administration, and decision making. As a student, I had experience in making decisions under the supervision of my mentor, but now, in my new role as a staff nurse, I was completely accountable for my decisions.

Accountability in nursing is a multifaceted and complex issue, with key implications for the profession. It carries with it ethical and legal implications, as well as implications for patient care (Sorensen et al. 2009). Hollywood (2011) found, from her study, that accountability was a positive aspect for some newly qualified nurses and a negative aspect for others. Some newly qualified staff nurses found that professional account-ability provided them with a sense of ownership (Hollywood 2011), but the reality of professional accountability has also been known to have a significant effect on the tran-sition experience of newly qualified nurses, causing them anxiety and stress (Sorensen et al. 2009).

 Exercise

1. Consider the factors that might contribute to decision making for each of the following situations.
   (a) Management of time in the clinical area
   (b) Prioritizing care needs
   (c) Delegation
   (d) Drug administration
2. Identify resources that would provide professional support to the decision-making in each of the situations.

The qualitative research study carried out by Hollywood (2011) highlighted a high level of anxiety on the newly qualified staff nurses' part in relation to the responsibilities that came with their new roles and also the fear of making mistakes. The newly quali-fied nurse in the case study often felt self-conscious that she was slower than her colleagues in making decisions and completing tasks, which sometimes resulted in stress, because she found herself in an unfamiliar situation and was afraid of making the wrong decisions.

 Exercise

Identify the resources that could verify your understanding of how to carry out a particular skill. Discuss with your personal tutor whether they are realistic expectations in practice.

The types of resource that you may have identified will have included:

● Trust procedure manuals;
● experienced staff;
● national guidelines, such as those issued by the National Institute for Health and Clinical Excellence (NICE) and the National Patient Safety Agency (NPSA); and
● professional development workshops.

In my first two weeks, I struggled with low levels of self-confidence, and found it difficult to interact and seek support from senior staff, because I felt intimidated by their increased levels of knowledge and experience. This would fall under the sociocultural and developmental components of Duchscher's (2007) transition shock model. Duchscher (2008) found, from his studies, that newly qualified staff nurses found it ultimately devaluing to interact with senior staff whose behaviour reinforced hierarchical, rather than collegial, relationships, because they found it difficult to relate to these staff, and felt uncomfortable expressing their worries and concerns. On my first day, I was introduced to many staff nurses who worked on the unit. They were all very friendly and reassured me that I would be well supported, and would be able to ask anybody for help and support. Although the staff were all very friendly and supportive, I initially felt as though I wasn't a part of the team.

Levett-Jones and Lathlean (2007) describe this as 'belongingness'. Belongingness is defined as a personal experience that evolves in response to the degree to which an individual feels secure, accepted, included, valued, and respected by a group, that he or she is connected with or is integral to the group, and that his or her professional or personal values are in harmony with those of the group (Levett-Jones and Lathlean 2007). According to Maslow (1987), evidence suggests that people who are deprived of belongingness may experience low self-esteem. Anant (1967) further states that depression, anxiety, and increased stress may also be experienced, as well as a decrease in general well-being and happiness (Lakin 2003).

Research carried out by Levett-Jones et al. (2009) showed that a lack of belongingness from a student nurse's perspective may result in poor practice, motivation to learn, and future career decisions. This shows the severity of the consequences caused by deprivation of belongingness.

As I gradually became familiar with the practices and daily routines on the unit, I slowly started to become confident in my role as a staff nurse. I was also able to relate to the senior staff on the unit a lot better and felt comfortable in asking them questions, because they were all very approachable and were always applauding me for my development. My preceptors regularly had meetings with me, were always willing to teach me new knowledge and skills, and reassured me that they were there for me if I needed any extra support. This helped me to feel like I was valued and I finally felt a part of the team.

As I completed my preceptorship period, I felt confident in my role, and learned that I would always work as a safe practitioner as long as I worked within my

(Continued)

limitations and asked for help, advice, and support when needed. I now feel confident in making clinical decisions where appropriate and have the maturity to ask for help when I feel I'm out of my depth.

As I commenced my new role as a newly qualified staff nurse, I felt I was back in my first year at university again. This was because being a registered nurse was a completely new and unfamiliar experience for me. I therefore started again at level 1 of Steinaker and Bell's (1979) taxonomy as I approached my new experience as a registered staff nurse—but I quickly reached level 5 of the taxonomy as a result of the skills and knowledge that I'd gained as a student.

From this newly qualified nurse's experience, we can see that if a well-supported preceptorship programme is in place and a supportive nursing team is able to facilitate the newly qualified staff nurse's learning needs, a smooth transition from student nurse to staff nurse will be achieved. This has also been supported by Higgins et al. (2009).

Conclusion

This Chapter has described the newly qualified nurse's experience and critical reflection of practice. We can see the complexity of decision making in action, not only for the student nurse making the transition to newly qualified nurse, but also, as in all of the other three chapters in **Part 3**, in terms of personal development and growth in decision making as the nurse is exposed to various different experiences with patients, service users, carers, parents, and families. It is important as well, as we will see in **Chapter 13**, that learning to make decisions and ensuring that you have the prerequisite knowledge and skills does not stop on qualifying.

The preceptorship period to which this newly qualified nurse was exposed enabled her to build her confidence in decision making and continued to build on the competencies achieved on qualifying as a registered nurse. Her newly developing skills and knowledge enabled her to interact with these young parents in the care of their newborn baby, but also enabled her to work with them because of her growing understanding of what it might be like as an adolescent parent. Her ability to act as an advocate on their behalf with other health care professionals and to facilitate decision making was evidence of her role transition confidence.

We hope that you will be able to use the reflective sections and the activities to explore your own experiences with children, and their parents and families, and use this nurse's experience as an example for critically reflecting on and learning from your own decision-making skills in practice.

References

Anant, S. (1967) 'Belongingness and mental health: some research findings', *Acta Psychologia*, 26: 391–6.

Beauchamp, T. L. and Childress, J. F. (1983) *Principles of Biomedical Ethics*, 2nd edn, New York, Oxford University Press.

Bee, H. L. and Boyd, D. (2007) *The Developing Child*, Boston, MA: Pearson, Allyn & Bacon.

Benner, P. (1984) *From Novice to Expert: Excellence and Power in Clinical Nursing Practice*, Menlo Park, CA: Addison Wesley.

Biehl, M. and Halpern-Felsher, B. L. (2001) 'Adolescents' and adults' understanding of probability expressions', *Journal of Adolescent Health*, 28(1): 30–5.

Cagean, J. and Meier, P. (1983) 'Evaluation of a discharge planning tool for use with families of high-risk infants', *Journal of Obstetric, Gynaecologic and Neonatal Nursing*, 12: 275–81.

Chen, X. K., Wen, S. W., Fleming, N., Demissie, K., Rhoads, G. G., and Walker, M. (2007) 'Teenage pregnancy and adverse birth outcomes: a large population-based retrospective cohort study', *International Journal of Epidemiology*, 36(2): 368–73.

Child Development Institute (2011) 'Stages of social-emotional development: Erik Erikson', available online at <http://www.childdevelopmentinfo.com/development/erickson.shtml>

Clack, G. (2009) 'Decision making in nursing practice: a case review', *Paediatric Nursing*, 21(5): 24–7.

Clark, T. and Holmes, S. (2007) 'Fit for practice? An exploration of the development of newly qualified nurses using focus groups', *International Journal of Nursing Studies*, 44(7): 1210–20.

Cole, M. and Cole, S. R. (1993) *The Development of Children*, 2nd edn, New York: Scientific American Books.

Cole, M. and Cole, S. R. (2001) *The Development of Children*, 4th edn, New York: Worth.

Coyne, I. (1995) 'Parental participation in care: a critical review of the literature', *Journal of Advanced Nursing*, 21(4): 716–22.

Department for Education and Skills (2006) *Teenage Pregnancy Next Steps: Guidance for Local Authorities and Primary Care Trusts on Effective Delivery of Local Strategies*, Nottingham: DfES.

Department of Health (2001) *Seeking Consent: Working with Children*, London: Department of Health.

Department of Health (2006) *Every Child Matters in the Health Service*, London: Department of Health.

Duchscher, J. E. B. (2007) *Professional Role Transition into Acute Care by Newly Graduated Baccalaureate Female Registered Nurse*, Dissertation Abstracts International (DAI-B 68/10): AAT NR.32924.

Duchscher, J. E. B. (2008) 'Transition shock: the initial stage of role adaptation for newly graduated registered nurses', *Journal of Advanced Nursing*, 65(5): 1103–13.

Erikson, E. (1956) 'Erikson's eight stages of development', available online at <http://www.childdevelopmentinfo.com/development/erickson.shtml>

Glasper, A. and Richardson, E. A. (2006) *A Textbook of Children and Young People's Nursing*, London: Churchill Livingstone.

Gomes, S. (2010) 'Discharge planning and the community outreach service', in M. Meeks, M. Hallsworth, and H. Yeo (eds) *Nursing the Neonate*, 2nd edn, Chichester: Wiley Blackwell, pp. 345–57.

Gormley-Fleming, L. and Campbell, A. (2011) 'Factors involved in young people's decisions about their health care', *Nursing Children and Young People*, 23(9): 19–22.

Gutman, L. M., Brown, J., Akerman, R., and Obolenskaya, P. (2010) *Change in Wellbeing from Childhood to Adolescence: Risk and Resilience*, London: Institute of Education.

Health Development Agency (2007) *Teenage Pregnancy and Parenthood: A Review of Reviews*, London: Health Development Agency.

Higgins, G., Spencer, R. L., and Kane, R. (2009) 'A systemic review of the experiences and perceptions of the newly qualified nurse in the United Kingdom', *Nurse Education Today*, 30(6): 499–508.

Hollywood, E. (2011) 'The lived experiences of newly qualified children's nurses', *British Journal of Nursing*, 20(11): 661–71.

Huband, S. and Trigg, E. (2003) *Practices in Children's Nursing: Guidelines for Hospital and Community*, London: Churchill Livingstone.

Johns, C. (1994) 'Nuances of reflection', *Journal of Clinical Nursing*, 3(2): 71–5.

Johns, C. (2000) *Becoming a Reflective Practitioner: A Reflective and Holistic Approach to Clinical Nursing, Practice Development and Clinical Supervision*, Oxford: Blackwell Science.

Kohlberg, L. (1969) 'Stage and sequence: the cognitive-developmental approach to socialization', in D. A. Goslin (ed.) *The Handbook of Socialization Theory and Research*, 2nd edn, Chicago, IL: Rand McNally, pp. 347–480.

Lakin, J. (2003) 'Exclusion and role of non-conscious behavioural mimicry: the role of belongingness threat', Unpublished PhD thesis, Ohio State University, Columbus, OH.

Levett-Jones, T. and Lathlean, J. (2007) 'Belongingness: a prerequisite for nursing students' clinical learning', *Nurse Education in Practice*, 8(2): 103–11.

Levett-Jones, T., Lathlean, J., Higgins, I., and McMillan, H. (2009) 'Staff student relationships and their impact on nursing students' belongingness and learning', *Journal of Advanced Nursing*, 65(2): 316–24.

Major, D. A. (2010) 'Student nurses in transition: generating an evidence base for final placement learning-facilitation best practice', Unpublished MPhil thesis, University of Salford.

Mallik, M. (1997) 'Advocacy in nursing: a review of the literature', *Journal of Advanced Nursing*, 25(1): 130–8.

Maslow, A. (1987) *Motivation and Personality*, 3rd edn, New York: Harper and Row.

McLeod, P. (2008) 'Erik Erikson', available online at <http://www.simplypsychology.org/Erik-Erikson.html>

Mental Health Foundation (2011) *Children and Young People*, London: Mental Health Foundation.

Nursing and Midwifery Council (2008) *The Code: Standards of Conduct, Performance and Ethics for Nurses and Midwives*, London: NMC.

Nursing and Midwifery Council (2010) *Standards for Pre-Registration Nursing Education*, London: NMC.

O'Regan, H. and Fawcett, T. (2006) 'Learning to nurse: reflections on bathing a patient', *Nursing Standard*, 20(46): 60–4.

Peplau, H. E. (1952) *Interpersonal Relations in Nursing*, London: Macmillan Education.

Piaget, J. (1972) 'Intellectual evolution from adolescence to adulthood', *Human Development*, 15(1): 1–12.

Sorensen, E. E., Seebeck, E. D., Scherb, C. A., Specht, J. P., and Loes, J. L. (2009) 'The relationship between RN job satisfaction and accountability', *Western Journal of Nursing Research*, 31(7): 872–88.

Spano, S. (2003) 'Adolescent brain development', *Youth Studies Australia*, 22(1): 36–8.

Spence, K. (2000) 'The best interest principle as a standard for decision making in the care of neonates', *Journal of Advanced Nursing*, 31(6): 1286–92.

Spouse, J. (2001) 'Workplace learning: pre-registration nursing students' perspectives', *Nurse Education in Practice*, 1(3): 149–56.

Steinaker, N. and Bell, R. (1979) *The Experiential Taxonomy: A New Approach to Teaching and Learning*, New York: Academic Press.

United Nations Children's Fund (2000) *The UN Convention on the Rights of the Child*, London: UNICEF.

Warren, I. (2010) 'Developmental care', in M. Meeks, M. Hallsworth, and H. Yeo (eds) *Nursing the Neonate*, 2nd edn, Chichester: Wiley Blackwell, pp. 316–33.

Wolfe, D. A., Jaffe, P. G., and Crooks, C. V. (2006) *Adolescent Risk Behaviours: Why Teens Experiment and Strategies to Keep Them Safe*, New Haven, CT: Yale University Press.

Wyatt, J. (2010) 'Neonatal ethics', in M. Meeks, M. Hallsworth, and H. Yeo (eds) *Nursing the Neonate*, 2nd edn, Chichester: Wiley Blackwell, pp. 334–44.

Further Reading

Coyne, I., Neill, F., and Timmins, F. (2010) *Clinical Skills in Children's Nursing*, Oxford: Oxford University Press.

O'Brien, I., Duffy, A., and O'Shea, E. (2010) 'Medical futility in children's nursing: making end-of-life decisions', *British Journal of Nursing*, 19(6): 352–6.

Twycross, A. and Powls, L. (2006) 'How do children's nurses make clinical decisions? Two preliminary studies', *Journal of Clinical Nursing*, 15(10): 1324–35.

Useful Links and Resources

<http://standards.nmc-uk.org/PublishedDocuments/Standards%20for%20
pre-registration%20nursing%20education%2016082010.pdf>

Pages 40–48 of the NMC Standards (2010) cover competencies for children's nursing.

<http://www.euro.who.int/__data/assets/pdf_file/0017/102257/E81512.pdf>

The World Health Organization (WHO) website offers a range of documents related to the WHO Europe Children's Nursing Curriculum, of which this strategy document is one example, focusing on the decision-making processes in each of four case studies.

<http://www.nhs.uk/Tools/Pages/Toolslibrary.aspx?Tag=Child+health>

The NHS Choices website offers many resources related to the knowledge and skills required to underpin effective decision making in children and young people's nursing.

11

Decision making in adult nursing

Deborah Atkinson and Jane McGrath

The aims of this chapter are to:

- ➔ help you to understand why clinical decision making is an important element of nursing practice;
- ➔ consider the complexities of clinical decision making in the field of adult nursing;
- ➔ consider how to recognize the factors influencing clinical decision making in practice;
- ➔ provide a strategy to improve your clinical decision-making ability; and
- ➔ consider the importance of including the patient in the decision-making process, wherever possible (shared decision making).

Introduction

This chapter explores clinical decision making in the field of adult nursing practice. It draws upon the actual experiences of a third-year student nurse prior to qualifying as a nurse, to provide real-world examples of the types of decision that you, as a student nurse, will face whilst out on placement and once qualified. The case studies include learning exercises for you to complete, which aim to explore how you might have addressed the situation and made decisions. This will help you to develop skills for safer professional practice and to put the patient at the centre of your decision making.

The role of the nurse in decision making

The role of the nurse has grown significantly over recent years as a result of changes in health policy, enabling the nurse to take on far greater levels of responsibility, such as independent nurse prescribing and advanced levels of nursing practice. This has resulted in nurses working in an increasingly complex clinical environment. On a daily basis, nurses are required to make decisions in relation to the care that they provide and how they manage their individual workloads (Banning 2005). As such, clinical judgement is considered to be an essential skill (Tanner 2006). Nurses now have far greater independence over their decisions in clinical practice owing to the influence of the changing policy context (Thompson 2001). However, this level of independence brings increased responsibility to the nurse, who will be judged and held accountable for his or her actions. Nurses are frequently required to make decisions in practice, often with limited information available to them (Ellis 1997). This requires critical thinking and problem-solving abilities, which are important elements of student nurse education (Garrett 2005).

Clinical decision making is a highly complicated process, not yet fully understood, and there is considerable debate relating to its constructs and definitions evident in the literature (Shabban 2005). Furthermore, a variety of terms are used interchangeably within the literature referring to clinical decision making, which demonstrates a lack of consensus and may cause confusion: 'clinical judgement', 'clinical decision making', and 'clinical reasoning' are phrases used interchangeably to discuss and describe similar activity (Maharmeh 2011).

Consequently, there is a confusing array of theory, opinion, and terminology relating to the decision-making process (Buckingham and Adams 2000). Whilst a definition for 'clinical decision making' varies among authors, there is some agreement that the process involves a deliberate choice between a range of options and acting within this choice (Thompson and Dowding 2004). Nurses make a clinical decision based upon their initial assessment of a situation, using prediction to gauge the likely impact of that decision in the future (Shabban 2005), and are responsible and accountable for their decisions (Thompson 2001; Watson 1994). Clinical decisions may be based upon various types of knowledge, the sources of which have been the subject of considerable philosophical enquiry. The quest to understand the different types of knowledge within nursing continues, on the basis that there remains much to be discovered about the nature of nursing knowledge (Liaschenko 1998).

The initial nursing assessment relies upon the gathering and interpretation of patient data by the nurse using sophisticated cognitive processes to produce a communicable account of the patient's condition (Chase 1995). A decision can then be made based upon the judgement made at the time. An accurate nursing assessment and judgement of the situation are therefore critical to effective decision making. However, when we make decisions in our daily practice, we are influenced by many things. For example, we may be pressured to make a decision by the patient, a relative, or by a colleague. Many factors may exert some influence over our decisions. What is important for us to consider is that all of our decisions have consequences. We therefore want to be confident that the decision made will result in a positive outcome.

Effective decision making in practice is essential in order to improve clinical outcomes for patients, and to develop and improve our practice. There are many theories that have attempted to discover how and why we make decisions in clinical practice. However, exploring how and why we make certain decisions in practice can help us to learn from experience and to develop decision-making skills for the future. An important consideration for us, as nurses at all levels, is that the patient should be at the centre of all that we do. Wherever possible, we must involve the patient in the decision-making process and always act to ensure that the patient's best interests are preserved. Involving patients in the decision making relating to their care has been shown to improve patient outcomes (Bechel et al. 2000). The government has since published a White Paper (Department of Health 2010) that promises patients that they will be included in the decision-making process, enshrining the principle of 'no decision about me, without me'. Similarly, the Nursing and Midwifery Council (NMC) *The Code: Standards of Conduct, Performance and Ethics for Nurses and Midwives* (NMC 2008) demands that nurses and midwives collaborate with those in their care.

Case studies in adult nursing practice

Case study 11.1 depicts a commonly occurring event in a busy accident and emergency (A&E) department, but one that requires highly effective decision making from the clinical team in order to maximize the outcome for the patient. It highlights some major learning themes, including the concept of family-witnessed resuscitation (FWR), the breaking of bad news, and the emotional impact on family members, nurses, and patients when someone dies.

Case study 11.1 Decision making in the immediate situation

A third-year student nurse has begun placement in a busy A&E department. Today was her second shift and she was working with her mentor. Notice was sent by the ambulance service of a patient en route to the department in cardiac arrest. Afterwards, the student nurse writes up the situation that she faced, which is typical of the types of situation in which you could be involved during a clinical placement. (Similar experiences could also apply to students following the other field-of-practice pathways, who may be undertaking an elective placement or an 'exposure to other fields' spoke placement in an A&E department.)

(Continued)

Case study 11.1 (Continued)

The incident began when a call arrived in A&E announcing the imminent arrival of a patient in cardiac arrest, with an estimated arrival time of 1 minute. Immediately, urgent preparations began for the patient's arrival and the team began to assemble in readiness to respond. It was briefly explained to me what to expect and I was fully encouraged to be involved from the outset. This was my first experience of a resuscitation situation.

One of the nurses went with me to meet the ambulance. I held open the doors and helped with transporting the patient by stretcher; as I did so, I observed how all members of the team rushed into action, each with their own roles and responsibilities.

In the resuscitation room, the doctors and nurses worked well together as part of a team endeavouring to resuscitate the patient. The patient was subsequently intubated and chest compressions were then carried out continuously. Throughout these events, I ensured that I was not 'in the way' and stood at the side of the room in order to observe. Although I had undertaken basic life support training at university in preparation for such events on several occasions, I realized that the reality of cardiopulmonary resuscitation (CPR) in an emergency 'life or death' situation was very different from the calm, safe surroundings of a clinical skills laboratory, and I began to experience feelings of self-doubt and inadequacy. I didn't offer to help with the chest compressions until the senior nurse asked me to pass her a waters circuit. I was grateful for the opportunity to assist and, a short time later, I offered my help. I then began performing chest compressions whilst under the supervision of the qualified nurse.

The patient's son was very distressed in the waiting room and asked to be present whilst CPR was taking place. The son was then invited into the room during the resuscitation attempt of his mother. Whilst both doctors and nurses continued with the ventilation and chest compressions on the patient, her devastated son was crying and begging his mum not to die, and to hold on to life. He was clearly very distressed. The son's presence and his obvious desperation intensified what was already a highly emotional situation. Once again, I took the role of observer. I felt as though I should have shown him support or said words of comfort, but I simply observed and said nothing ...

Questions

Imagine yourself as the student nurse in this situation. Consider the following questions.

1. Why did the student not get involved in the resuscitation attempt at first?
2. What happened to prompt the student to get involved?
3. What are the factors that may have influenced this decision?
4. What could the student have done to improve her decision making for the future?
5. What helps you to make decisions in practice?
6. Have you identified any learning points from the case study?

(Continued)

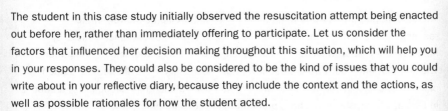

Case study 11.1 (Continued)

Issues to consider

The student in this case study initially observed the resuscitation attempt being enacted out before her, rather than immediately offering to participate. Let us consider the factors that influenced her decision making throughout this situation, which will help you in your responses. They could also be considered to be the kind of issues that you could write about in your reflective diary, because they include the context and the actions, as well as possible rationales for how the student acted.

(1) Knowledge, skills, and prior experience

The case study illustrates a 'life and death' situation in the A&E department. The student nurse involved had only ever practised basic life support in a controlled classroom environment. The real-life situation was a very different experience, with consequences for the patient.

When we are faced with a clinical decision-making situation, one of the first considerations that we make as nurses is whether we have the required level of knowledge and skill to perform the nursing intervention.

In this instance, the student nurse felt confident with the underpinning rationale and had practised the skill required on previous occasions, but not in a real-world situation. It was her lack of actual experience of the situation that prevented her from actively participating in the resuscitation attempt. The speed of events prevented the opportunity to discuss this with her mentor before the patient arrived. However, if the situation had not been so urgent, the student could have discussed this prior to attending the patient. The student had practised the skills required and also knew the underpinning theory of CPR. It was only her lack of experience that prevented her from volunteering to join in at the outset.

(2) Confidence

The student nurse was new to the A&E department. She was in awe of the clinical team around her, and their level of skill and confidence in managing this critical situation. The student felt that she was less able than the other team members.

The lack of prior experience in resuscitation caused to student nurse to lack confidence in her ability to resuscitate the patient. The other team members were all very accomplished in their field of practice and familiar with the resuscitation scenario. They also clearly worked well as a team, and were all clear about their individual roles and responsibilities during the resuscitation attempt. As a newcomer to the department, the student nurse had not yet established her place within the team and was concerned that her actions might hinder those of the other team members.

(Continued)

Case study 11.1 (Continued)

(3) Fear and apprehension

The student nurse was worried that if she were to participate actively in the resuscitation, she might make a mistake or be in the way of the other clinicians, hindering the resuscitation and making the outcome less favourable for the patient. The fact that other staff were present with the necessary skills allowed the student an element of choice. However, if the student had been alone in the presence of a patient in cardiac arrest, she would have probably behaved quite differently.

- If a patient had suffered cardiac arrest and the student nurse was alone, her decision making would probably have been very different. It would have been far quicker for her to make the decision and her options would be limited.
- Ultimately, if the student were to have opted not to perform CPR in this situation, the patient would have died without urgent help from another member of staff.

The student's lack of experience and confidence made her apprehensive and fearful, asking herself 'What if...?' And yet the student nurse knew that her experience and confidence would not improve unless she grasped the opportunity to learn from the clinical situation in which she was involved. This opportunity was essential for her to gain practical skills experience for the future.

> The situation felt surreal, and I was in awe of everyone knowing their role, rushing around in an acute situation ... I felt frustrated with myself for not taking the opportunity to offer to participate and to take over performing chest compressions ...

The student overcame her fear and offered to participate in the resuscitation attempt. This was prompted by the senior nurse involving the student in the rescue, which occurred when the student was asked to pass a piece of equipment from the trolley. At that point, the student made a conscious decision to get involved because she:

- felt valued;
- was overcoming her fear; and
- recognized an important opportunity to gain experience.

The student understood the importance of gaining authentic experience whilst under the supervision of others. This would provide the opportunity to learn from others, as well as a chance to practise the skills previously learned in a controlled environment.

The senior nurse had included the student in the situation and this felt like an invitation to participate. Being included in the team demonstrated that the student was accepted by the other clinicians as a professional with a valuable contribution to make.

The student was able to overcome her fears of inadequacy because there was sufficient support and supervision available to her. A supportive environment is essential for inexperienced staff to develop their clinical skills and to develop

(Continued)

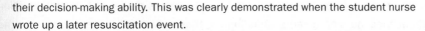

Case study 11.1 (Continued)

their decision-making ability. This was clearly demonstrated when the student nurse wrote up a later resuscitation event.

This time, I reacted totally differently. I felt focused and confident, and I felt able to become involved immediately. Because I'd already been on placement in the area for a few weeks, the environment felt familiar and I was also familiar with the other staff, which helped. On this occasion, I felt able to become involved from the beginning, helping to prepare the area before the patient arrived. Once the patient had arrived in resus. I made myself available to help out where I could and performed chest compressions along with another staff member, alternatively, for 30 minutes. I then asked if I could be involved with the family, and observed breaking bad news and helping to support the relatives. The initial experience gave me the confidence to do that, and I think my self-doubt and feelings of inadequacy were an initial hurdle that the original experience helped me to overcome.

The clinical decision-making processes illustrated in **Case study 11.1** follow the 'hypothetico-deductive model' (see **Chapter 1**). This model processes information made by the nurse during the initial assessment of the situation and generates tentative hypotheses for the various decision-making options available at the time. The decision-making process is somewhat laboured, with careful consideration being given to all of the known possible outcomes. The main problem with this, of course, is that, as an inexperienced student or newly qualified nurse, it is not possible for you to know all of the possible decisions or the influence of other variables on a decision.

As a nurse becomes more proficient in recognizing specific risks, managing certain situations, or practising particular skills, the clinical decision-making process becomes easier and less evident. It also becomes more difficult for the nurse to articulate. At this point, the decision-making process has become more intuitive (Benner 1984) or based upon tacit knowledge gained through practical experience (Eraut 2000). This ability has been largely associated with expertise in nursing practice.

As you progress through your nursing education and eventually qualify as a nurse, it will be necessary for you to practise independently, to analyse situations, to make assumptions, and to solve problems through the use of critical thinking, clinical judgement, and decision making (Gabr and Mohamed 2011). Problem-based learning, or enquiry-based learning, is a strategy that can be used to help with clinical decision making in practice. Traditionally used in the educational setting, it requires a collaborative approach between the student and teacher or mentor, and requires the student to take the initiative for defining his or her own learning goals and to become a self-directed learner, rather than to be passive in the learning environment.

Problem-based learning has been shown to influence learning outcomes positively, including the development of logical and critical thinking ability, problem solving, and decision making (Yuan et al. 2008). These skills are extremely important for nurses, who ought to aspire to be lifelong learners, being responsible for self-directed learning throughout their nursing careers. Additionally, these skills will benefit nurses in the constantly changing clinical environment, helping them to make decisions in atypical clinical situations.

The following activities will ask you to use a problem-based or enquiry-based learning approach relating to the real-life clinical case studies that are included in this chapter. These case studies presented are intended to generate critical thinking and self-directed learning, empowering you by allowing you to decide what you need to learn.

 Exercise

Read through **Case study 11.1** again. The following questions follow a problem-based learning approach.

1. What knowledge would be essential for you, as a student, to participate in CPR for the patient?
2. Where might you locate this essential information?
3. What other knowledge or information would be useful, but not essential in making the decision?

 Top Tips

When faced with a clinical decision in practice, consider what knowledge you *already have* relating to the presenting problem or issue. Then, work out what other *essential* information you require to make your decision safe. Once you have this information, give some thought to what *additional information* might be beneficial, but not essential. This information can be researched at a later point in time, during home study or discussed with your mentor. It is useful to jot down any gaps in knowledge in a notepad for future reference.

This strategy adopts a 'problem-based learning' or problem-solving approach to making decisions in your clinical practice, which incorporates the learning that you have acquired as a student nurse and builds upon that knowledge. Being 'reflective in action' (Schon 1983) highlights the areas of your knowledge that require additional learning.

Useful information resources include libraries and the Internet—but be sure that electronic resources are reliable. Some useful websites that you may wish to use to locate research evidence for practice include:

- <http://www.bestbets.org>
- <http://www.cochrane.org>
- <http://www.medicine.ox.uk/bandolier>
- <http://www.nelh.nhs.uk>

In answering the first exercise, you should have noted the following.

1. *Essential knowledge*—Practical skills experience in performing chest compressions and rescue breaths in a cardiac arrest situation (either in a classroom or clinical skills laboratory-based situation, or with a genuine patient) is essential knowledge for the student to make the decision to participate.

2. *Important knowledge*—Knowledge relating to the various pieces of equipment that may be used in the CPR situation is important, so that the student can assist with passing the equipment to team members and so that the team is safe during the CPR attempt. This is especially important when a defibrillator is being used.

3. *Additional knowledge*—Understanding the individual roles and actions undertaken by each of the team members is useful for the student, so that he or she can adopt one of these roles at a later stage. This might include being the 'script', who records the timings of events as they unfold; it might be running through an intravenous (IV) infusion in readiness to connect to the patient's IV access; or it might be knowing how to manage the patient following a successful resuscitation.

⊕ Exercise

Write down what knowledge, skills, and experience you have relating to CPR, using the following questions as a guide.

- What essential knowledge do you have?
- What essential knowledge do you need?
- What else would be important to learn about?
- What other information would be useful for the future?

Now, let us think about the decisions made by the student nurse later that day relating to the death of the patient and the care of the grieving relative.

Case study 11.2 Decision making during and after the situation

The patient's son was very distressed in the waiting room and asked to be present whilst CPR was taking place. The son was then invited into the room during the resuscitation attempt of his mother. Whilst both doctors and nurses continued with the ventilation and chest compressions on the patient, her devastated son was crying and begging his mum not to die, and to hold on to life. He was clearly very distressed. The son's presence and his obvious desperation intensified what was already a highly emotional situation. Once again, I took the role of observer. I felt as though I should have shown him support or said words of comfort, but I simply observed and said nothing.

Eventually, a decision was made by the doctor for the resuscitation team to stop CPR, because it was deemed unsuccessful. It was at this point that the staff nurse broke the sad news to the patient's son. The staff nurse very sensitively turned to him and explained that, unfortunately, the resuscitation attempt hadn't worked, and how very sorry she was. The incident was extremely emotional for all involved. Throughout the experience, I was supported by the nurses, and was asked several times if I had any questions and how I felt.

At the end of the resuscitation attempt, the patient's son was offered the opportunity to take time to reflect in a quiet room, was supported at all times by the nursing staff, and was given the opportunity to speak to the senior doctor to help him to come to terms with recent events and to ask any questions that he may have.

I helped one of the nurses to make the patient comfortable and then moved the patient in a bed to the prayer room, remaining there with her relative. It was a very difficult experience to watch the son's very early stage of acceptance, whilst trying to come to terms with the loss of his mother.

Questions

1. In this instance, the student seems to be disappointed that she did not offer the relative any words of comfort during the witnessed resuscitation. Why do you think this is?
2. Adopting the same approach as previously, consider what knowledge and information is needed to make a decision about whether or not to comfort the relative.
   (a) What knowledge is essential?
   (b) What knowledge is important?
   (c) What would be additional useful information?

➡ Top tips

As you become more familiar with using problem-based or enquiry-based learning to help with decision making in practice, you might think of these three questions as

- What must I know?
- Should I know ... ?
- Could I know ... ?

Being able to comfort a distressed patient or relative is fundamental to nursing care. While death is inevitable for everyone at some stage, health care professionals often find it very difficult to break bad news and to deal with grief. In **Case study 11.2**, the student felt unable to offer the distressed relative any words of comfort during the resuscitation attempt. This may have been the first time that the student had been in the presence of a distressed relative. The student may have felt ill equipped to answer some of the questions that the relative may ask.

It is important to understand that your management of the situation during this type of traumatic event may have a lasting memory for the relative. Showing empathy and giving support is extremely important. However, it is also important to be able to identify cues and understand body language from the relative or patient, which invites you to show that empathy.

➕ Exercise

1. Have you been involved in comforting a patient or relative, or been present during the breaking of bad news?
2. What did you learn from the experience and what do you think might be helpful to other students?
3. What are your fears, if any, about being in this type of situation and how can you address these?
4. What research evidence is available relating to this area of practice?

Use these questions to guide your reflection of a situation (see **Chapter 4**) and write down your experience in your reflective diary or as a specific 'significant event', which can help you to achieve some of the NMC competencies (NMC 2010).

Our ability to make decisions in practice is largely reliant upon our prior knowledge and experience.

➲ Top Tips

It is good practice to have a 'debrief' with your mentor towards the end of each shift. Spend a few minutes discussing what went well for you during the shift, and identify areas in which you feel that additional learning and experience is needed to improve your knowledge and decision making for the future. Your mentor can then facilitate an action plan to address these areas of learning with you. The debriefing process is an opportunity for you to reflect on your practice and the decisions that you have made. This will help you to identify the areas of practice in which you are confident, as well as those in which you feel additional support may be needed. This promotes the taking of responsibility for your own learning.

We will now consider decision making in another context, with which some of you may already be familiar.

Case study 11.3 Decision making: the need for knowledge of the diagnosis and its implications for the patient

An elderly woman had been admitted into the A&E department with a possible stroke. The patient was alert and talking, and had relatives present. The patient was waiting to be transferred to the acute medical unit for a full assessment, but had already been in the department for almost three hours and was now feeling hungry and thirsty. The relatives asked if I could fetch their mother a cup of tea.

Question

What should the student nurse do in this situation?

1. Fetch the patient a cup of tea.
2. Ask her nurse mentor whether the patient is able to have a cup of tea.
3. Tell the patient and relatives that it is not yet permissible for the woman to eat or drink anything.
4. Explain to the patient and relatives that a swallowing assessment would be required before she could have anything to eat or drink, to prevent any risk of aspiration.

Issues to consider

What are the risks faced by patients who have been diagnosed with a stroke? The Stroke Association (**<http://www.stroke.org.uk>**) offers a range of information for patients that explains what to expect from their assessment in hospital.

(Continued)

Case study 11.3 (Continued)

Did you consider the following areas of care?

- Pressure area relief and assessment
- Venous thrombo-embolism prevention
- Prevention of aspiration and effect of a stroke on the swallowing mechanism
- Blood glucose management in stroke
- Maintaining hydration
- Maintaining nutrition
- Patient education
- Personal care
- Promoting independence

You may have identified many other aspects of care in which clinical decisions would be required. This demonstrates the complexities of clinical decision making in practice for nurses. Wherever possible, refer to national guidance or robust research evidence to assist you with clinical decisions. Where practicable, involve your patients in the decision-making process. For this elderly patient and her relatives, however, the most immediate decision was that related to her being able to have a cup of tea. The possible responses of the student nurse may all be considered appropriate, except the first—that is, fetch the patient a cup of tea. This would be a decision that may appear logical, in that the patient is feeling thirsty, but would in fact be contradictive of her care needs at that time: the patient has not yet had a full assessment, including assessment of her swallowing ability.

If you suggested that you would check with your mentor, this shows that you are aware that if you are unsure, you are required to check with a qualified nurse.

Either of the other two responses indicate that you may have sought guidance from your mentor as to what to say to the relatives, but also that you would offer them an evidence-based rationale for this.

Using the available evidence base to support the decision-making process is essential in order to be able to give a rationale for the decisions that we make (see **Chapter 3**). Research evidence can be published in peer-reviewed journals or reported in other non-peer-reviewed journals, and is incorporated into the development of national guidance (as is available through the Stroke Association, for example). The difficulty for professionals in practice is keeping pace with the available literature that informs our practice. Additionally, we require the skills to critically appraise the quality of published work in order to evaluate the strengths and weaknesses of a study (Holland and Rees 2010).

As nurses, it is necessary to ensure that our practice is current, as dictated by the NMC Code (NMC 2008), which sets out the standards of conduct, performance, and ethics for nurses and midwives. **Box 11.1** is an extract from the Code.

Box 11.1 Extract from the Nursing and Midwifery Council Code (2008)

Provide a high standard of practice and care at all times

Use the best available evidence

35 *You must deliver care based on the best available evidence or best practice.*

36 *You must ensure any advice you give is evidence-based if you are suggesting health care products or services.*

37 *You must ensure that the use of complementary or alternative therapies is safe and in the best interests of those in your care.*

Keep your skills and knowledge up to date

38 *You must have the knowledge and skills for safe and effective practice when working without direct supervision.*

39 *You must recognize and work within the limits of your competence.*

40 *You must keep your knowledge and skills up to date throughout your working life.*

41 *You must take part in appropriate learning and practice activities that maintain and develop your competence and performance.*

(NMC 2008: 6)

Similar statements can be found in the NMC's *Guidance on Professional Conduct for Nursing and Midwifery Students* (NMC 2011) and it is important that you familiarize yourself with this document, which guides your practice as a student nurse and will inform your decision making in practice.

 Exercise

Access the Guidance online at **<http://www.nmc-uk.org/Documents/Guidance/NMC-Gui dance-on-professional-conduct-for-nursing-and-midwifery-students.pdf>**
Ensure that you are familiar with the requirements that it outlines.

These professional standards are intended to safeguard the public in our care. We therefore have a professional responsibility to keep up to date with new evidence and to incorporate this into our practice and decision making.

Exercise

Consider the following questions.

- How do you keep up to date with new evidence?
- How do you know whether the evidence is reliable?
- How do you include new research evidence into practice?

 Top Tips

A useful way of incorporating new research evidence into your clinical practice is to develop a 'journal club'. This is a forum that brings peers together at a dedicated time to consider newly published literature relating to practice. The journal club members review relevant publications together, appraising the methodology, results, and implications for practice of various studies. The group is usually facilitated by a senior team member in the practice environment or by a tutor at university. As a student nurse, this format of group learning is maybe something with which you are already familiar.

The following are some ideas for making a journal club successful.

1. Focus on the current real patient problems of most interest to the group.
2. Bring questions, a sense of humour, and some snacks and drinks.
3. Distribute (and redistribute) the time, place, and topics for the meeting, and the roles of the group members, in advance.
4. Bring enough copies for everyone of the papers for review, including both the 'article of the week (or month)' and a backup article.
5. Keep handy multiple copies of quick (one-page) quality appraisal tools.
6. Keep a log of the questions asked and answered by the group.
7. Finish with the group's agreed conclusions and develop an action plan for disseminating the knowledge acquired.

Conclusion

This chapter has focused on the clinical decision-making process in the field of adult nursing practice. It has provided a number of real-life clinical case studies for you to consider, using a problem-solving, enquiry-based learning approach to help in developing clinical decision-making skills. These case studies can assist all students across the four fields of practice, and the questions asked can be applied to a variety of experiences as you progress along your chosen pathway to become a registered nurse. They clearly demonstrate how the evidence base to decision making (see **Chapter 3**) and reflection on learning (see **Chapter 4**) is important as a generic learning outcome that can then be applied in a field-specific context. Decision making of any kind (see **Chapter 1**) is fundamental to the practice of nursing in any context and field of practice. (See **Chapters 9**, **10**, and **12** for further examples.) It is a skill that we would encourage you to develop from the outset of your programme, and upon which you should continue to build as you qualify as a nurse and take on the responsibility of being an accountable practitioner.

References

Banning, M. (2005) 'A review of clinical decision making: models and current research', *Journal of Clinical Nursing*, 17(2): 187–95.

Bechel, D. L., Myers, W. A., and Smith, D. G. (2000) 'Does patient-centred care pay off?', *Joint Commission Journal of Quality Improvement*, 26(7): 400–9.

Benner, P. (1984) *From Novice to Expert: Excellence and Power in Clinical Nursing Practice*, Menlo Park, CA: Addison Wesley.

Buckingham, C. D. and Adams, A. (2000) 'Classifying clinical decision making: a unifying approach', *Journal of Advanced Nursing*, 32(4): 981–9.

Chase, S. (1995) 'The social context of critical care judgement', *Heart and Lung*, 24(2): 154–62.

Department of Health (2010) *Equity and Excellence: Liberating the NHS*, London: Department of Health.

Ellis, P. A. (1997) 'Processes used by nurses to make decisions in the clinical practice setting', *Nurse Education Today*, 17(4): 325–32.

Eraut, M. (2000) 'Non-formal learning and tacit knowledge in professional work', *British Journal of Educational Psychology*, 70: 113–36.

Gabr, H. and Mohamed, N. (2011) 'Effect of problem based learning on undergraduate nursing students enrolled in nursing administration course', *International Journal of Academic Research*, 3(1): 154–62.

Garrett, B. (2005) 'Student nurses' perceptions of clinical decision making in the final year of adult nursing studies', *Nurse Education in Practice*, 5(1): 30–9.

Holland, K. and Rees, C. (2010) *Nursing: Evidence-Based Practice Skills*, Oxford: Oxford University Press.

Liaschenko, J. (1998) 'The shift from the closed to the open body: ramifications for nursing testimony', in S. Edwards (ed.) *Philosophical Issues in Nursing*, London: Macmillan Press, pp. 11–30.

Maharmeh, M. (2011) 'Coronary care nurses: developing an understanding of the decision making process in acute situations', Unpublished PhD thesis, University of Salford.

Nursing and Midwifery Council (2008) *The Code: Standards of Conduct, Performance and Ethics for Nurses and Midwives*, London: NMC.

Nursing and Midwifery Council (2010) *Standards for Pre-Registration Nursing Education*, London: NMC.

Nursing and Midwifery Council (2011) *Guidance on Professional Conduct for Nursing and Midwifery Students*, London: NMC.

Schon, D. (1983) *The Reflective Practitioner: How Professionals Think in Action*, London: Temple Smith.

Shabban, R. Z. (2005) 'Theories of clinical judgement and decision making: a review of the theoretical literature', *Journal of Emergency Primary Health Care*, 3(1–2), available online at <http://www.jephc.com/full_article.cfm?content_id=192>

Tanner, C. A. (2006) 'Thinking like a nurse: a research-based model of clinical judgement in nursing', *Journal of Nursing Education*, 45(6): 204–11.

Thompson, C. (2001) 'Clinical decision making in nursing: theoretical perspectives and their relevance to practice—a response to Jean Harbison', *Journal of Advanced Nursing*, 35(1): 134–7.

Thompson, C. and Dowding, D. (2004) 'Awareness and prevention of error in clinical decision making', *Nursing Times*, 100(23): 40–2.

Watson, S. (1994) 'An exploratory study into a methodology for the examination of decision making by nurses in the clinical area', *Journal of Advanced Nursing*, 20(2): 351–60.

Yuan, H., Kunaviktikul, W., Klunklin, A., and Williams, B. A. (2008) 'Improvement of nursing students' critical thinking skills through problem-based learning in the People's Republic of China: a quasi-experimental study', *Nursing and Health Sciences*, 10(1): 70–6.

Further Reading

Burton, R. and Ormrod, G. (2011) *Nursing: Transition to Professional Practice*, Oxford: Oxford University Press.

Garrett, B. (2004) 'Student nurses' perceptions of clinical decision making in the final year of adult nursing studies', *Nurse Education in Practice*, 5(1): 30–9.

Holland, K. and Roxburgh, M. (2012) *Placement Learning in Surgical Nursing: A Guide for Students in Practice*, Edinburgh: Bailliere Tindall Elsevier, esp. pp. 41–58.

Useful Links and Resources

<http://standards.nmc-uk.org/PublishedDocuments/Standards%20for%20
pre-registration%20nursing%20education%2016082010.pdf>

Pages 13–21 of the NMC Standards (2010) cover competencies for adult nursing.

<http://www.advancedpractice.scot.nhs.uk/legal-and-ethics-guidance/what-is-ethics/et
hical-frameworks-and-decision-making.aspx>

The NHS Scotland Advanced Practice Toolkit website offers a number of resources related to ethical decision making.

<http://www.ukcen.net/index.php/ethical_issues>

The UK Clinical Ethics Network offers information and a number of case studies in relation to ethical issues.

12

Decision making in learning disability nursing

Sue Hart and Eva Scarlett

The aims of this chapter are to:

➔ explain the value base underpinning decision making with people who have learning disabilities;

➔ provide examples from practice of how and why decisions are made, and the thought process involved; and

➔ draw attention to some of the particular challenges that you may encounter when making decisions for and with people who have learning disabilities.

Introduction

This chapter focuses on exploring decision making in the learning disability nursing field of practice. Previous chapters have covered the background about decision making, the principles, tools, and the use of evidence, as well as the way in which decision making fits in with the Nursing and Midwifery Council (NMC) *Standards for Pre-Registration Nursing Education* (NMC 2010) and competencies. The content of these early chapters and learning will help you to build your understanding of the issues when applied particularly to learning disability nursing skills in practice.

This chapter also follows those addressing decision making in mental health nursing, children and young people's nursing, and adult nursing. This 'separating out' of the fields of practice is helpful to give particular clarity and focus to issues relevant within them. It is, however, equally important to remind you that these apparently clear-cut distinctions between the disciplines are not necessarily reflected in practice, and that clients and patients do not always fit neatly into these artificial 'boxes'. People with a learning disability have a right to equal treatment from registered nurses in adult and mental health settings, and children and young people with learning disabilities should expect the same standard of care as their typically developing peers. The NMC's *The Code: Standards of Conduct, Performance and Ethics for Nurses and Midwives* (NMC 2008: 3) reminds us that 'You must not discriminate in any way against those in your care' and that 'You must treat people as individuals and respect their dignity'. So, whatever your chosen future field of practice, please read on, because when people with learning disabilities require nursing, they are—and always will be—your responsibility too.

Case study 12.1 has been chosen intentionally to highlight the partnership working and decision making that can go on between adult nurse specialists and learning disability nurses.

Value-based decision making

 Exercise

You work on a busy surgical ward. Two male patients, both aged 48, have been admitted this afternoon, for elective haemorrhoidectomy surgery tomorrow. Mr A is a full-time university lecturer married with one child; Mr B is single and packs bags at his local supermarket for 8 hours a week and, with three others, is resident in a supported living service. Mr B is known to the local community learning disability team, since he was referred by his general practitioner (GP) for dietary and hygiene advice following several bouts of chronic constipation.

Think about the nursing decisions made for each of these patients at the following points:

- prior to admission;
- at pre-assessment clinic;
- on admission;
- during admission;
- before discharge; and
- at follow-up.

Are the same decisions going to be made for each? If not, how and why might they differ?

The underpinning value base of decision making in learning disability nursing today is best understood with brief reference to the past. It is in recent memory for many service users that 'home' was a long-stay hospital ward or villa, which, despite the best efforts of nursing staff, would invariably be managed along quite regimented lines. It was simply not possible to manage large numbers of people in such settings *and* offer genuine choices, shared decision making, and individualized care. (See Goffman 1961, and Korman and Glennerster 1990, if you want to understand this background in more detail.)

With *deinstitutionalization*, the widespread 'warehousing' of people ceased and enabled the establishment of many small-scale community-based residential services. These aimed to provide a much more 'ordinary life' (Kings Fund 1980). The most forward-thinking learning disability nurses and service managers of the time also used this opportunity to rethink their overall service ethos, based on ideas such as O'Brien's (1987) five accomplishments and developing caring practices with the new idea of enabling more 'person-centred' care (Brechin and Swain 1987). A key tenet of these newly developing services was to enable choice and decision making.

O'Brien's (1987) idea was that choice for people with learning disability meant 'a basic and fundamental right to have autonomy and control over decisions about all aspects of life, day-to-day issues, and major life events' (summarized by Thomas and Woods 2004, p. 70). The beginnings of a focus on person-centred care ensured that it was more likely than in previous regimes of care that individual choices, preferences, and decisions were, if not always put into practice, at least being considered. *Valuing People* (Department of Health 2001), the cross-government policy that gives a direction to learning disability services for the twenty-first century, stressed people's right to self-autonomy and self-determination.

Previous chapters will have noted that good decision making is ideally a partnership between the nurse and patient or client. In learning disability nursing, enabling as much choice and decision making as the person is capable of is a fundamental skill that is practised numerous times daily, and often over a long term—not only for an admission to a ward or unit for treatment and discharge. Learning disability nurses make decisions about how best to support people with learning disabilities to make their own choices, to identify their own preferences, and, as far as they are able, to make their own decisions.

Decision making in Practice

Please note that, in all of the following case studies, the person's name and other identifying characteristics have been changed significantly to preserve confidentiality. However, in each case, the decisions needing to be made and the practice underpinning this are based on real-life situations.

Case study 12.1 illustrates the decision making involved when a woman known to the community nursing team is admitted to hospital.

Case study 12.1 Alina's story

Alina is in her mid 20s and lives in a high-rise flat in an industrial town in the north of England. She lives independently, with community support worker input for 4 hours a week. Alina has a 3-year-old daughter, who now lives full-time with her father, Dan, Alina's former partner. Dan does not have a learning disability. Alina has a good relationship with Dan and still sees her daughter, but accepts that she is unable to look after her full-time. Alina is close to her extended family, especially since her mother's death two years ago. Alina has one brother, who also has a learning disability and lives in a residential service.

Alina has been known to her local community team for people with learning disabilities (CTPLD) since a referral from her GP. He was concerned about Alina's use of crack cocaine (a highly addictive drug) and felt that she needed some healthy lifestyle advice.

In an incident that Alina cannot remember, she was badly bitten by a stray dog and taken as an emergency to her local hospital. A routine blood test on admission caused concern and later investigations confirmed that Alina had acute lymphoblastic leukaemia, the same disease that had caused her mother's death. Alina was admitted to the oncology (cancer) ward and, following a case discussion, it was agreed that the cancer specialist nurse would make contact with the CTPLD.

Questions

1. What issues does this scenario raise both for Alina and for the nursing and medical staff in the hospital?
2. For what reasons may the team have decided to involve the CTPLD?
3. Try to predict what some of the key decisions may be in a case like this.

Issues to consider

The learning disability nursing team were told that Alina's condition was life-threatening and that she needed to be offered the opportunity to start chemotherapy as soon as possible. For this to be successful, she needed to avoid the risk of infection and nursing her in a side room in hospital for the six-week duration of the treatment was recommended. When the cancer nurse and, later, the oncologist had explained this to Alina, they were not certain that she understood the implications, because she made several slightly odd and unconnected comments, which caused concern about her understanding.

Decisions

(1) Appropriate referral

The CTPLD had to decide whether it felt that this was an appropriate referral. When it was agreed that it was, the team had to decide which nurse was best placed to work with Alina in these circumstances. Should a team member who was also a registered

(Continued)

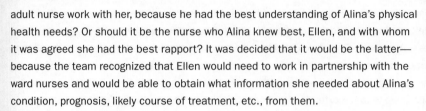

Case study 12.1 (Continued)

adult nurse work with her, because he had the best understanding of Alina's physical health needs? Or should it be the nurse who Alina knew best, Ellen, and with whom it was agreed she had the best rapport? It was decided that it would be the latter— because the team recognized that Ellen would need to work in partnership with the ward nurses and would be able to obtain what information she needed about Alina's condition, prognosis, likely course of treatment, etc., from them.

(2) Determining the urgency

Was this a routine referral or was it time-sensitive, requiring immediate action? The team manager discussed the case as a one-to-one with Ellen, the allocated nurse, and it was decided that she should go to the hospital that afternoon as a priority. This decision was made for several reasons. Ellen knew that Alina was likely to be very frightened in the hospital on her own, and that, often in such circumstances, she would refuse food and drink. Ellen knew that her presence would be a reassurance for Alina and that, as long as she was not nil by mouth, they could have a drink together. Ellen could also take a bottle of water for Alina: she would always drink from her own bottle, even if she was refusing liquid from others. The referring nurse had also said that a case meeting was going to be held that afternoon with the consultant present, and Ellen knew that this would be a good opportunity to understand the clinical picture and what she would need to do to support Alina through the process. Finally, it was clear to Ellen and her manager, from what the referring nurse had said, that acute lymphoblastic leukaemia was a life-threatening condition and that acting without delay was essential.

(3) Planning the interventions

On the 20-minute bus journey to the hospital, Ellen reflected on the events of the morning, from the referral to what she had heard so far, and then used her notebook to jot down in shorthand some of the questions that she wanted to ask and some of the actions she thought may be needed. She would use these notes as prompts for herself, but they would be necessary only if these areas did not come up in discussion. Forward planning in this way is good practice and helps to ensure that nothing is forgotten.

Ellen also decided that it was best to meet with the medical and nursing team first, rather than to go straight to see Alina, again for various reasons: she did not want to arrive at Alina's bedside and then immediately be drawn away; Ellen also knew that Alina may not like the idea that 'people' were talking about her when she was not present; and finally Ellen herself would be more confident to work with Alina when she had a better understanding of the current situation. She had to avoid doing or saying anything that could be misleading. Alina was likely to ask 'How long do I have to stay in here

(Continued)

Case study 12.1 (Continued)

for?' or 'Am I going to die?' It was important that Alina could trust Ellen, and this was going to be best achieved by the two spending time together and Ellen helping Alina to understand her condition (Marsham 2011). Before the meeting, Ellen did not have a good sense of the answers to these questions and needed to decide how best to communicate information to Alina.

(4) Meeting the cancer ward nursing and medical team

The consultant oncologist summarized the circumstances to date and how the diagnosis had been found by accident, as a result of blood tests following the dog bite. She stressed that Alina was 'lucky' in this respect, because it meant treatment could begin soon, and this in turn meant a much better chance of full recovery. She explained that she had told all of this to Alina, who had at first shed some tears and then made some 'odd' responses, as if in shock. She had repeated 'parrot fashion' over and over again several of the phrases the doctor had used. She had not displayed this behaviour before, during her admission. The consultant had been suddenly very concerned about Alina's mental state and agreed with the team that input from 'someone who knows Alina' was urgent.

What if Alina had not been known to the local CTPLD team and had been unable to give details of a next of kin or friend? What action might the hospital have taken then and who could it have involved?

(5) Decisions made at the hospital meeting

- Alina's learning disability and 'odd' response had called into question her mental capacity to agree to the proposed treatment, and it was decided that this needed to be assessed before she could give consent.

- It was acknowledged that Alina probably had not fully understood the implications of what the oncologist had said to her. Ellen advised the team that she could use accessible resources (such as Books Beyond Words) and information from **<http://easyhealth.org.uk>** to ensure that Alina understood.

- It was decided that this intervention would be essential if Alina were to make an 'informed decision' about her treatment.

- It was decided that if Alina were found to not have mental capacity to agree to treatment, a 'best interest' meeting would be called.

(6) First meeting with Alina

Ellen went to see Alina in her side room on the ward immediately after the meeting. It was about six months since they had last met, and Ellen had decided that she at first must 'catch up' with Alina and prompt her to talk. To the untrained eye, such

(Continued)

Case study 12.1 (Continued)

'chatting' may seem casual and unstructured; to a learning disability nurse, this is the foundation of an assessment. Through these exchanges, Ellen was assessing Alina's mood, her level of anxiety, and her appearance (had she been self-caring), and whether she understood that she was in a hospital or, conversely, if she made no reference to this fact. In these circumstances, an experienced learning disability nurse would not necessarily use a 'formal' assessment tool. Rebuilding a therapeutic relationship and trust (after a gap of six months) is not always most effectively accomplished by the filling in of forms and the answering of tick-box questions. Giving time, listening, reassuring, and comforting were Ellen's first goals. Showing empathy and care were essential to this process. After an hour, it was clear that Alina had some understanding of being in hospital and that her 'blood had gone wrong'. She seemed to think that she was going to have an operation and was not happy about this. Ellen was able to reassure Alina that this was not the case, but she needed to have some medicine to make her 'blood better'. At this point, Ellen felt that Alina had been given enough information, and that sitting with her and encouraging her to eat the supper that had just arrived would be the most effective intervention. Ellen said that she would return the next day to chat more. Her decision was rooted in the need to:

● find useful accessible resources and to plan to do a mental capacity assessment the next day; and

● allow Alina time to absorb the conversation that they had just had and to be fresh the next day to think more about her condition.

(7) Second meeting with Alina (next day)

Ellen's first task was to remind Alina of her visit the previous day and to assess how much she could recall of their conversation. Based on this assessment, Ellen knew that the resources she had brought with her would be helpful to go over the important areas again. Using simple language and pictures, Ellen was convinced that Alina understood 'blood' and 'chemotherapy'. Importantly, she also understood that her illness was very serious and that, without treatment, she may die. Alina understood that it was the same illness that had led to her mother's death. She said: 'I don't want to die.' Ellen also noticed that, at times in the conversation, Alina was displaying the behaviour described by the oncologist and repeating Ellen's words 'parrot fashion'. A useful technique in these circumstances is to rephrase the question and then to ask the person to repeat back his or her understanding of what was said. This intervention showed that Alina had a good basic understanding of the illness and proposed treatment. Ellen told Alina that it was time to invite the junior doctor to her room so that written consent to treatment

(Continued)

Case study 12.1 (Continued)

could be given. With staff nurse Kumar present, Ellen questioned Alina to show that she could:

- understand the information given to her;
- retain that information long enough to be able to make a decision;
- weigh up the information available; and
- communicate the decision.

These principles are central to the Mental Capacity Act 2005 and Alina's responses confirmed that she understood enough to be able to give consent to her treatment. It was apparent that Alina knew the implications of not being treated (that is, that she may die) and that she was clear in her desire that this should not happen.

Case study 12.1 has shown how professionals work together to support the person to make decisions and also how important it is for a person to be assessed for his or her capacity to make important decisions for himself or herself, assisted by accessible literature (see **<http://easyhealth.co.uk>**). Alina went on to have the chemotherapy and stayed in hospital for this over a period of six weeks. The team advised that she remain as isolated as possible from others to minimize the risk of infection, and Alina found this the most difficult part of the process. She is now home and doing well.

Key issues to consider when making decisions with people who have learning disabilities

Before the next two case studies, the chapter will highlight some areas for particular consideration in this field of practice.

Concept of *informed* decisions

It is good practice always to ensure that patients give informed consent, for example, prior to a surgical procedure. The Mental Capacity Act 2005 Code of Practice 2007 outlines how people should be helped to make their own decisions. The concept of 'enough' information is important here. It is not a kindness to unduly worry a person with a learning disability about a possible risk when, in reality, the chance of this occurring is very slim (such as the risk of bowel perforation during a routine colonoscopy).

The use of alternative forms of communication, sign-supported language, such as Makaton, pictures, and other accessible resources can be helpful in aiding understanding. Excellent examples of resources to support decision making around health needs are available online at **<http://easyhealth.co.uk>**

When a person lacks capacity to make an important decision on his or her own, a 'best interest' meeting of the professionals and others close to the person is often used to agree, and record, what is felt to be the best outcome for the person involved.

Ethical dilemmas

The Mental Capacity Act 2005 makes provision for people who have capacity to make decisions that professionals must honour, *even if it is believed that they are unwise*. If a person with a mild learning disability is assessed as capable of consenting to treatment, he or she has a right to refuse as well as to agree to what is being offered.

Assessing the risk of people with learning disability to undertake a particular activity (such as, after transport training, to travel alone into town on a bus) is a key aspect of work in this field of practice. In this context, careful decisions need to be made with the person involved to ensure that the fine balance is reached between ensuring that people are safe (that is, the duty of care) and enabling as much independence as possible.

Family–person tensions

Many parents of those with learning disabilities strive for them to have lives that are as 'normal' as possible. For example, parents have been known to 'fight' education authorities to ensure that their son or daughter has mainstream education, and afterwards to aim for them to go to college and get a job. Others take the view that people with learning disabilities essentially need care and protection, ideally sheltered from the 'rough and tumble' of everyday life. Once he or she is an adult, this latter view may run counter to what the person wants for his or her own life. In this instance, decision making can be fraught, often with professionals placed in the role of facilitator or chief negotiator. Tensions can run deep as professionals weigh up the risks and act as advocates for their clients, as well as honour their duty of care to the person and responsibility to their own employer, and *at the same time* acknowledge the concern of family, who love their son or daughter and simply want to keep him or her safe. Decision making in such cases involves carefully balancing the competing demands and delicate negotiation between the parties, or relationships can easily become fractured or even break down.

Types of decision

How a decision is made depends on what it is. Some decisions are simple—tea or coffee, jam or marmalade—and can be thought of as a simple choice between two or more possibilities, with no major implications resulting from the decision made. Many people with even quite severe learning disabilities are able to exercise such choices through 'eye pointing' or a nod of the head. This contrasts with the more complex decisions for a person with a learning disability who has *mental capacity*, for example to decide whether or not to have a sexual relationship, to move to another service provider, or, because he or she is frightened of the anaesthetic, to say 'no' to treatment for an operable and potentially life-saving malignant tumour on his or her lung. Here, good learning disability nursing practice would be to take all practical steps to maximize the person's ability to make the decision. We would do this by giving relevant information, in a format that the person can understand, and supporting him or her to weigh up what might be the advantages and disadvantages of making a particular decision, until the person comes to his or her own conclusion.

Longer term planning and decision making

Some decisions, such as those above, are required to be made in the short term. Other decisions set a path for a person to follow, a goal to achieve, or a dream to fulfil.

Consider, as an example, Helen, who is 19 and has autism, and who is about to go to Florida with her parents to swim with dolphins. The decision was made with Helen, her family, her health care support worker, and the community registered learning disability nurse during a person-centred planning meeting two years ago (Sanderson 1997). Helen's team used a planning tool called 'Maps' (Forest et al. 1997). This approach has its focus on a 'dream' that the person has and a 'desirable future'. With support, Helen was able to communicate that she has a dream of living in a flat with her friend, Suzie, having a dog, working in Sainsbury's stacking shelves, or being on the confectionery counter. She also said that she wanted to go swimming with dolphins. She is still working towards the other goals, with a possible tenancy coming up soon and 'job training' starting when she gets back from the US. Without the forward thinking and the decisions made at the time, with Helen at the centre of the process, she may not have moved forward at all.

Case study 12.2 concerns a man who has a mental health need, as well as a learning disability.

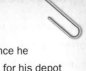

Case study 12.2   Dinesh's story

Dinesh has been known for a short time to the local community nurses since he moved out of his family home into a flat. He is seen once every two weeks for his depot medication (a long-acting antipsychotic intra-muscular injection, Depixol). Although enjoying his new-found 'freedom', it seems that Dinesh is also making some questionable decisions for himself, and causing his mother and support worker a lot of concern.

Dinesh is a young man in his early 30s who has a mild learning disability and a history of mental health needs, including drug-induced psychosis and hypomania. He has been known to the learning disability team for six months since he moved into his own flat in an inner-city shared house with four others, who also have learning disabilities. Living in the city gives Dinesh easy access to local shops, cafés, and activity centres, such as the gym and the library. Dinesh receives minimal input from a support worker twice a week, and enjoys his personal space and independence, having previously lived with his mother and younger sister. He values being able to do what he wants without 'permission' and having a place of his own.

For the past ten days, Dinesh has begun to experience dystonia (particularly facial tics), which he knew could be a result of his current medication Depixol (British Medical Association and the Royal Pharmaceutical Society of Great Britain 2007), an antipsychotic treatment. Dinesh contacted the team to explain what was happening to him and a visit was arranged by his community nurse.

In order to decide what action to take, the nurse initially referred to Dinesh's case notes to see if this side effect had been a problem before, and if so, how it had been managed. There may not always be notes available, for example with a new referral to the team. In this case, further information would need to be gathered from the service user or their carer during an initial assessment.

The visit to Dinesh was held at his home and, with his agreement, had been planned to coincide with the end of his support worker appointment, so that James, who knows Dinesh very well, would be able to provide additional background information.

The community nurse began by encouraging Dinesh to explain his concerns; he talked about the 'tics' and other muscle spasms, and how he felt that they were embarrassing and made him feel self-conscious. The nurse reassured Dinesh that he was probably right about the cause and said that he would talk with Dinesh's psychiatrist later that day, and ask for an assessment of the current medication and exploration of alternative options.

When working with people with learning disability, it is not unusual to make a home visit for one reason only to find, when there, that there are other concerns to attend to that are at least as important as, and often which are more pressing than, the original reason. The decision here was to find out how could the nurse have the greatest effect on Dinesh and work with him in a person-centred way to meet his needs. The decisions were all made jointly with Dinesh, James, and the consultant psychiatrist.

(Continued)

Case study 12.2 (Continued)

It was following this prompt that Dinesh mentioned that he had a rash on his buttocks, which he thought might be a result of the medication injection site. He agreed that the nurse could look and it was immediately obvious that the actual injection site was not the cause. In discussion, Dinesh said that he did sweat a lot and wondered if this was the cause. The nurse advised Dinesh to keep the area clean and dry, and to wait for a week to see if the rash improved; if no improvement was seen, he should go with James to see his GP.

Prompted by James, Dinesh then told the nurse that he regularly smokes cannabis, which he had been doing since he left home. The nurse used this opportunity gently to tease out more information about Dinesh's habit and was relieved to hear that he did not smoke 'hard drugs', such as heroin or crack. It was a concern, however, that Dinesh admitted owing about £20 to the drug dealer. He also expressed an awareness of the negative issues surrounding smoking the drug and said that his mother wishes he would stop.

Question

Consider the dilemma that this declaration about taking drugs raises for the community nurse. The NMC requires us to keep information confidential—but this is criminal behaviour. How would reporting this to the police affect the nurse–patient relationship?

Issues to consider

In this case, the nurse discussed the matter with the psychiatrist and they noted in Dinesh's file that they agreed not to report at this stage, but that they may need to reconsider the decision at a later date.

They agreed that Dinesh accepting the help that he needed and staying as well as possible was the primary goal. A reason for reconsidering the decision could be if there were a significant escalation in the behaviour, evidence of selling drugs, or evidence of Dinesh being harmed in anyway by other drug users.

Decisions

(1) Dystonia

It was decided to ask Dinesh and his support worker, James, to come to a psychiatry outpatient appointment, with the community nurse and consultant. Dr Jones reviewed Dinesh's mental health and had no concerns apart from the facial twitching. It was decided to change the medication to Aripiprazole, which has fewer side effects (British Medical Association and the Royal Pharmaceutical Society of Great Britain 2007). However, this would have to be in an *oral* medication. Later, the nurse explained to

(Continued)

Case study 12.2 (Continued)

Dinesh and James how the medication could be placed in a 'blister pack', with the days and times clearly marked, in order to remind him to take the tablet. This would also make it easier for staff to monitor whether the medication was being taken.

(2) Drug use awareness

The next home visit would include an explanation in more detail about the potential dangers of taking drugs. Although Dinesh had expressed awareness of some dangers, he also seemed to believe that because 'nothing bad' had happened to him so far, it was unlikely to happen to him in the future. It was important that Dinesh be made aware of the possible harms of illegal drug taking, for example the negative side effects such as paranoia and nausea, and also the effect that it can have on his mental health.

(3) Drug use cessation

The next decision centred on the interventions that could be used to support Dinesh to stop smoking cannabis, especially because this may improve the sweating and by doing so improve his rash. It would also create a healthier lifestyle and one without risk of getting into trouble with the police. The nurse decided that it would be helpful to provide Dinesh and James with details of a drug smoking cessation helpline or website, and to encourage them to engage.

(4) Personal safety

The professionals agreed to encourage the repayment of the £20 as soon as possible and to counsel Dinesh about the danger of owing money to drug dealers.

(5) Positive social stimulation

It had been apparent, during the discussion, that Dinesh seemed to smoke cannabis when he had nothing else to do. Was this because he was bored? Dinesh was a very sociable individual, but his current associates tended to expose him to poor lifestyle choices. Supporting him to get new friends by indulging in hobbies or activities might encourage a new social group. Dinesh showed considerable enthusiasm when talking about other things that he could do to relax, such as swimming. A referral was to be made to an exercise consultant who worked with the team.

(6) Finances

Dinesh also seemed open to the thought of part-time employment. Dinesh had expressed a desire to go on a holiday and said he had never flown on an aircraft. Planning a holiday could be possible if Dinesh were to save the money he was spending on drugs (around £20 per week) and also being paid for work. Work also would help Dinesh to feel part of his local community, in a meaningful and rewarding way, and to keep himself busy in order to alleviate his boredom and cannabis smoking. His understanding of money would need to be assessed and possibly he may benefit from a

(Continued)

Case study 12.2 (Continued)

course aimed at building on his skills. This also would help to alleviate his boredom and encourage him to meet other people.

(7) Monitoring progress

At the fortnightly appointments to have his depot medication, the rash on Dinesh's bottom could be monitored, along with his current level of drug taking to see if it was rising or falling after the suggested interventions.

The final case study illustrates aspects of the decision-making process and actions that follow an initial referral of a young woman with severe learning disability to a CTPLD.

Case study 12.3 Kylie's story

Kylie, who is 17 years old, arrived in England from Canada a few months ago with her mother and brother. She has severe learning and physical disabilities. She walks with a broad-based, ataxic gait, with her hands often in the high guard position. She can also weight bear in a standing position. She cannot speak. Kylie has epilepsy and dysphagia (a disorder of swallowing). She can be prone to having seizures while eating.

Kylie's mother is a corporate development manager for an investment bank. Kylie's brother Leroy is 13 years old. He does not have a learning disability and attends a local mainstream school.

Kylie has been enrolled in a special educational needs school in the local area. As a result of the demanding nature of her job, Kylie's mother, who is not married, employed a nanny whilst in Canada, to support Kylie's needs with eating, drinking, and all of her personal care, and to give mobility assistance—because Kylie has a fear of falling, which can bring on her seizures.

The plan is that Kylie will be in England for four years. She is living here with her mother and brother, and her care is now being managed by her mother and two part-time agency carers are filling in for the moment until the Canadian nanny gets a work permit for the United Kingdom.

Issues to consider

The initial referral came from the deputy head at the school and was made by a telephone call to the community team leader. It was standard practice in this team for

(Continued)

Case study 12.3 (Continued)

anyone new to the area to be referred for assessment. This referral was also made as a result of an increase in Kylie's seizure activity. She had been having one seizure every five weeks on average when she was in Canada; since moving to the UK, she had been experiencing up to two seizures per week. The school reported that Kylie's mother was finding it difficult to manage (especially with taking Kylie out and also using the bathroom, owing to the risk of falling, which could bring on a seizure). The team met to decide how best to respond to this referral.

Deciding in a community learning disability team who should take the new referral

All learning disability teams will have standard procedures that must be followed, of which the following are an example.

   All new referrals come into a central point and then are passed on at a weekly meeting to the person best able to meet the needs. This decision is made entirely on the grounds of the nursing needs of the person, such as advice about behaviour, or health needs, such as the management of seizures or incontinence, etc. In some instances, CTPLDs employ social care professionals, as well as health care specialists. Here, a case was to be allocated within the team depending on the need for nursing *or* social care. Social care needs may involve housing, advice about benefits, or access to local leisure facilities. It is often the decision of the team leader how important, or even urgent, an issue is and this is communicated when the case is allocated.

   Kylie's case was allocated to a case manager with a nursing background in order to deal with the health needs—specifically, her epilepsy—and concerns about her weight and dysphagia, and Kylie's mother was contacted by telephone to arrange an appointment. The case manager was accompanied to the visit by a student nurse.

   Deciding where to carry out the assessment is important and it was agreed that home would be best in this case, because any issues to do with the home environment could be explored at the same time. Because there is often a need to gather extensive information, this is easier done in surroundings in which the family is most comfortable. To ensure that all topics are covered, it is good practice to draw up an agenda at the beginning of the meeting. This approach helps to foster a sense of partnership working with the person and his or her family, and suggests a shared agenda, rather than a professional dominating what happens.

Actions

With Kylie's mum's agreement, an initial assessment was carried out. This assessment tool had been developed by the local team and was accompanied by a health assessment. The aim was to gather enough information about the individual and his

(Continued)

Case study 12.3 (Continued)

or her family circumstances in order to determine what support needs he or she has in terms of health and social care. (An ideal outcome would be that a person is healthy and independent, and requires no additional support, but it was obvious in this case that this would not be the result.)

The initial assessment gathered information about Kylie's health, her abilities, and her needs. The information gathered soon highlighted that her younger brother had been 'helping out' with some aspects of his sister's care, at present, because Kylie's usual nanny had not yet arrived from Canada and the agency carers did not know Kylie very well. It was of some concern to hear that Kylie's brother was doing a considerable amount of hands-on care while her mother was not at home.

Decisions

(1) Sibling role as carer

An on-the-spot decision was made to highlight this as a serious issue. It needed to be approached immediately with sensitivity and tact in order to avoid offending the parent, whilst ensuring that the rights of the 'carer child' are met. It was also important not to damage the relationship between the siblings. Kylie's mother seemed genuinely to agree that it should not be the responsibility of a young teenager to look after his sister, but felt that there were no other options because of the pressures of her job and the absence of the nanny. She was reassured that the assessment is designed to determine the level of support needed in order to provide adequate care.

Sibling carers are not uncommon in the family of someone with a learning disability. In this case, the demands of the mother's job meant that she was out early in the morning and back late in the evening. With only part-time agency support, this actually left the brother to get Kylie ready for her school day and then to go on to school himself. Inevitably, this would have an impact on his school work, social life, and well-being. Under the Children's Act 1989, Kylie's mother has parental responsibility until Kylie reaches the age of 18, after which time she will be the responsibility of the local authority. Kylie's mother agreed to employ additional support to remove responsibility from Kylie's younger brother until the nanny arrived from Canada.

(2) Safety in the bathroom/occupational therapy referral

Kylie's falls had happened during personal care in the bathroom, because of the configuration of the room and lack of 'holding' places. The assessors observed Kylie in the bathroom, as her mother demonstrated how she was supported through her personal care routine. It seemed apparent that the placing of hand rails in three places that Kylie could grab would significantly reduce the risk of falls, which in turn would

(Continued)

Case study 12.3 (Continued)

reduce the risk of a seizure. It was decided to make an urgent referral to occupational therapy to assess the home and bathroom.

(3) Stabilizing the epilepsy

The referral had been prompted by the head teacher as a result of the increase in seizure activity and this obviously suggested that an appointment with a neurologist needed to be made, possibly for an electro-encephalogram (EEG), but also for a review of the anti-convulsant medication. This referral needed to come through the family's GP. It was a surprise to find that Kylie had not yet been registered with a GP and the assessors highlighted this as an urgent action for her mother. This is because the GP is the 'gatekeeper' within health care and many other referrals for Kylie would have to be progressed in this way. Kylie's mother agreed to register her with the GP.

(4) Carer needs

The initial assessment was also designed to highlight any particular needs for the carer. In this case, the assessment brought up the issue of the Canadian nanny's visa and the mother's frustration that it seemed to be taking so long.

(5) Future needs and transition

Kylie had multiple and complex needs, which were currently being met through professionals based within her school. She was seeing the speech and language therapist (SALT), who was supporting her with her communication needs. There were future plans for Kylie to learn Makaton. The SALT was also monitoring her dysphagia. This swallowing disorder can lead to coughing when the sufferer eats, because food enters his or her airways as a result of an inability to chew effectively. This can lead to chest infections. Kylie also had twice-weekly physiotherapy to assist with her mobility, which were aiming to increase her range of movements.

When young people with learning disabilities reach the age of 17, they are at the point of 'transition' from children's to adults' services. Because Kylie had so recently arrived in the UK, there were as yet no plans in place for her to move onto college, or to consider future adult service provision. It was decided that, to ensure the continuity of current therapeutic inputs, it was essential to make immediate referrals for adult service SALT and physiotherapy.

(6) Preparing Kylie and her family for the transition

A decision would need to be made about how best to do this. When she transferred to adult services, Kylie would access the help that she needs through the local authority and health service. This can be a challenge for individuals if they have been used to having all of their needs met in one place. Kylie would now have to meet new professionals, probably at different locations; she would have to get used to a whole

(Continued)

Case study 12.3 (Continued)

new set of people involved in her life. It is important to prepare for this as much as possible to make the transition smooth.

When Kylie's mother was next telephoned to review the progress of her actions, she explained that she had been unable to register Kylie with a GP because she had not had the time. Two further phone calls produced the same result and it became clear that this was an issue, because of the mother's job leaving her no time to commit to an appointment with the doctor. After some insistence, Kylie's mother eventually made an appointment to register Kylie with a GP. Later, again because of time constraints related to her job, Kylie's mother did not want to return to the GP to discuss the epilepsy and then also have to take another day to attend the appointment with the neurologist.

The decision now revolved around how to approach the mother, because previous efforts to encourage her to register Kylie with a GP had been unsuccessful. Regrettably, this meant changing tack and approaching her mother in a much more authoritative manner, pointing out the consequence (in this instance, a possible referral to a safeguarding team) if she were to fail again to register Kylie with a GP. This tension unfortunately meant that the relationship between her mother and the nursing team was significantly affected. The mother disengaged from working with the allocated case manager to support her daughter and contact with the team was kept to an absolute minimum. Often, calls or emails were not returned. This led to an increased workload for the team, because they would have to chase information or try to get it from outside agencies. However, in these circumstances, the need for Kylie to attend a neurology appointment was much more important than maintaining the relationship with Kylie's mother. When finally contact was made with the mother, she said that she had decided to make an appointment with a private neurologist in order to cut out the initial appointment with the GP. Kylie was to be sent the following week.

Outcome for Kylie and her family

The school has reported that Kylie's seizure activity has reduced. This could be a result of settling in to a new environment. It also reports that she is interacting well within the classroom environment and is well liked by her peers. As yet, neither the school nor the community team has received any notification from Kylie's mother regarding the outcome of the neurology appointment. It would be ideal to have this information to keep on record for future reference, but because the neurologist is private and Kylie's well-being seems to have improved, the team is less concerned about this than might otherwise have been the case. Kylie's nanny has now arrived from Canada, which means her mother can continue working and her brother no longer has the responsibility of providing Kylie's care. The transition process is ongoing and the actual transition will not happen until Kylie is 18 years old, at which point information will be retrieved from the school health professionals and passed onto the adult health care team.

The Nursing and Midwifery Council Standards (2010) and competencies

The chapter has illustrated through case studies how and why learning disability nurses make decisions with service users. It is impossible, within the confines of one book chapter, to explore all aspects of decision making across all of the field-specific competencies for learning disability nursing. Instead, we will focus on how some of the issues that we have explored in this chapter will facilitate learning to achieve one set of NMC Standards (NMC 2010) and one domain.

'Domain 3: Nursing Practice and Decision Making' (NMC 2010: 35–7) outlines the requirement that this aspect of competency be met in order to achieve registration. The following example competencies will show briefly how they link with practice. As a student nurse, you should consider each of these and how different your decision-making skills are from those of the qualified nurses working with people who have learning difficulties.

- *Competence 1.1* (NMC 2010: 35) stresses the need to respond to all people who come into the care of learning disability nurses. The case studies showed the diverse range of activity of learning disability nurses and how they draw on various techniques to ensure that needs are met.
- *Competence 3.1* (NMC 2010: 36) refers to nurses working in partnership and also the use of individual care plans for continuity of care. The case studies showed partnership working with medical professionals, a support worker, a special school, and a consultant psychiatrist. The competence also advocates a structured person-centred approach to any care, agreed in partnership with service users and carers, and other professional services and agencies. The case studies and activities will enable you to work towards achieving this competence.
- *Competence 5.1* (NMC 2010: 36) refers to the need to make plans for people's well-being and, most importantly, 'to facilitating equal access to all health, social care and specialist services'. Think back to **Case study 12.2** and recall how a request for help for one issue uncovered a range of other needs. With Dinesh's full engagement, a detailed plan was made to address the concerns and to help to redirect Dinesh to more positive lifestyle choices. In this case, a third-year student nurse working with the registered nurse was able to commit to a series of weekly meetings to provide fairly intensive input for Dinesh, with good results.
- *Competence 8.1* (NMC 2010: 36–7) refers to partnership working with families and transition of services. **Case study 12.3** draws attention to the reality that, sometimes, it is challenging to engage families and that professionals have to remain focused on the necessary outcomes in order to meet the duty of care to the individual. Although it did not go into detail, this case study also made reference to the transition to adult services on which Kylie would embark when she reached the age of 18.

Conclusion

Oi! It's My Assessment! was published by People First (1994), a self-advocacy group for people with learning disabilities. The aim of this booklet was to give information to people about community care, care management, and assessment that 'nobody has bothered to tell you'. It gave the message to people being assessed that they had a right to be given information, to make decisions about their care, their lives, and their health.

It is no longer helpful to think of learning disability nurses only as *caring* for the people with whom they work. Many people with learning disabilities do not want to live a life passively receiving care dictated by professionals and to be shut away from wider society. Most want to be enabled to lead lives with the maximum independence that they can achieve, and planning for this starts with the rights to be heard, to be taken seriously, and to be supported to make decisions. Current students of learning disability nursing should become the leaders of the future for this important and exciting development in this field of practice, because it will be up to *you* to lead the change, to make essential decisions for practice, and to make the difference.

References

Brechin, A. and Swain, J. (1987) *Changing Relationships: Shared Action Planning with People with a Mental Handicap*, London: Harper and Row.

British Medical Association and the Royal Pharmaceutical Society of Great Britain (2007) *British National Formulary No. 54*, London: BMJ Publishing Group.

Department of Health (2001) *Valuing People: A New Strategy for Learning Disability for the 21st Century*, Cm 5086, March, London: Department of Health.

Forest, M., Pearpoint, J., and Rosenberg, R. L. (1997) *All My Life's a Circle: Using the Tools— Circles, Maps and Paths*, 2nd edn, Toronto, ON: Inclusion Press.

Fovargue, S., Keywood, K., and Flynn, M. (2000) 'Participation in health care decision making by adults with learning disabilities', *Mental Health and Learning Disabilities Care*, (3)10: 341–4.

Goffman, E. (1961) *Asylums: Essays on the Social Situation of Mental Patients and Other Inmates*, Harmondsworth: Penguin.

Kings Fund (1980) *An Ordinary Life*, London: Kings Fund Centre.

Korman, N. and Glennerster, H. (1990) 'Changing attitudes to institutions', in N. Korman and H. Glennerster, *Hospital Closure*, Maidenhead: Open University Press, pp. 7–20.

Marsham, M. (2011) 'An exploration of community learning disability nurses' therapeutic role', *British Journal of Learning Disabilities*, 40(3): 236–44.

Nursing and Midwifery Council (2008) *The Code: Standards of Conduct, Performance and Ethics for Nurses and Midwives*, London: NMC.

Nursing and Midwifery Council (2010) *Standards for Pre-Registration Nursing Education*, London: NMC.

O'Brien, J. (1987) 'A guide to life style planning: using the activities catalogue to integrate services and natural support systems', in B. W. Wilcox and G. T. Bellamy (eds) *The Activities Catalogue: An Alternative Curriculum for Youth and Adults with Severe Disabilities*, Baltimore, MD: Paul Brookes, pp. 104–10.

People First (1994) *'Oi, It's My Assessment!' People First*, London: King's Cross.

Sanderson, H. (1997) 'Person centred planning', in B. Gates (ed.) *Learning Disability: Toward Inclusion*, Edinburgh: Churchill Livingstone, pp. 301–23.

Thomas, D. and Woods, H. (2004) *Working with People with Learning Disabilities. Theory and Practice*. London: Jessica Kingsley Publishers.

Further Reading

Gates, B. and Barr, O. (2009) *Oxford Handbook of Learning and Intellectual Disability Nursing*, Oxford: Oxford University Press.

Grant, G., Ramcharan, P., Flynn, M., and Richardson, M. (2010) *Learning Disability: A Lifecycle Approach*, Maidenhead: Open University Press.

Race, D. (2012) *Learning Disability: A Social Approach*, London: Routledge.

Useful Links and Resources

<http://standards.nmc-uk.org/PublishedDocuments/Standards%20for%20
pre-registration%20nursing%20education%2016082010.pdf>

Pages 31–39 of the NMC Standards (2010) cover competencies for learning disabilities nursing.

<http://www.easyhealth.org.uk>

The best available website for accessible health information, including videos and free downloadable guidelines.

<http://www.scie-socialcareonline.org.uk>

Social Care Online is a useful source of information about social care.

<http://www.talktofrank.com>

Frank is a website offering confidential advice about drugs.

Decision making for professional practice

PART 4

In keeping with the theme of continuing personal and professional development once qualified as a nurse, the final chapter will bring together the threads of decision making for professional practice and, in particular, decisions affecting the student's transition to 'newly qualified nurse'. It will provide guidance on how to develop effective decision-making skills to engage in the preceptorship period once qualified. Being a qualified nurse brings with it significant responsibilities and accountability, and therefore you will need to ensure that you remain aware of why you are making decisions and, of course, of when to make 'the right decisions at the right time and in the right way'. The responsibility and accountability of the registered nurse will require that future decision making must be based on the best possible evidence, as well as continuing education in relation to patient care, and personal and professional development.

13

Decision making for transition to registration and preceptorship

Sarah Ratcliffe and Joyce Smith

The aims of this chapter are to:

- explore the skills required for delegation, challenging others, and prioritizing decisions;
- discuss what the impact of transition from student nurse to qualified nurse will have on how you make decisions;
- consider issues of accountability in decision making; and
- consider decision making in the preceptorship period as a newly qualified nurse (registrant).

Introduction

This chapter will explore and discuss issues that may impact on your transition from third-year student nurse to newly qualified nurse (registrant). The issues that will be explored include delegation skills, challenging others, accountability, and prioritizing skills. Case studies will be included that will help you to consider how to respond in some situations that you may encounter. There are no right or wrong answers, but it is important to reflect on the many ways in which decision making occurs in terms of how you might act in certain circumstances. (See **Chapters 9, 10, 11,** and **12** for illustrations from actual practice situations.)

Based on the case studies described in the chapter and on the experience of the authors, top tips will be offered to help you to consider a range of options to deal with the identified problems.

It is hoped that the chapter will help you to plan key goals to achieve in your final placement, and to identify specific developmental goals to facilitate your transition to registered nurse and during your preceptorship experience.

Transition

'Transition' can be described as a challenging process that involves moving through a period of uncertainty from a familiar to an unfamiliar role. It is defined by Kralik et al. (2006: 323) as 'a passage from one life phase, condition, or status to another', often linked with a life-changing event. However, Meleis et al. (2000) state that change does not necessarily result in a transition and in fact change, according to Bridges (2003), is situational, whereas transition is psychological. Transition is a natural progression throughout life and, even though it can be actively sought and positive, it may be stressful as a result of psycho-social alterations (Brown and Olshansky 1997).

Bridges (2004: 4) describes transition as being 'composed of three stages: an ending, a neutral zone and a new beginning'. The first step is letting go, or ending, a past or former self; the next step, the neutral zone, is identified as a critical point for psychological readjustment; the final step is a new beginning. Bridges (2003) discusses fear of the unknown within the neutral zone, a stage of being in-between the end of the old and the beginning of the new. You probably experienced the process of transition when you first started the pre-registration nursing programme after moving from your previous role or employment.

....

⊕ Exercise

Reflect on your experience of the very first day of your new programme and the first stage of your journey to becoming a qualified nurse. What was your main concern on that day? If you had an occasion to write down your reflections in that day, re-read them and consider how you now feel about the last stage of your journey and becoming a qualified nurse. Write these feelings down in your reflective diary and you can read these again when you begin your next role as a qualified nurse in practice.

....

The impact of transition on nursing students has been explored periodically during the last three decades. In her seminal work, Kramer (1974) describes transition as a 'reality shock' and it is she who is credited with recognizing the impact of the transitional process on the newly qualified nurse. Many recurring themes have emerged since this work indicating that the impact of transition on nursing students and newly qualified nurses has remained constant throughout nursing's social, political, and educational changes. The transition from the academic setting, the *known*, to the clinical setting, the *unknown*, has been described by Duchsher (2009) as 'transition shock'. In addition, a comparative study of two cohorts of nursing graduates, undertaken in 1985 and 1998, revealed a feeling of unpreparedness for their new role, which they found stressful (Gerrish 2000). Similar studies involving pre- and post-registration students have identified inadequate preparedness with feelings of stress, anxiety, and uncertainty (Deasy et al. 2010).

Warne and McAndrew (2008) discuss this preparedness in relation to self-awareness, and suggest that there is an area between knowledge and knowing called 'not knowing', which has the potential to challenge our emotions or compromise and provide strength. Thus transition is a complex process that depends on insight and understanding of self, an insight into our own self-awareness, and therefore ultimately informs our nursing practice. Transition is inextricably linked to the self and identity, and how it may be affected by disruption (Kralick et al. 2006; Young et al. 2004).

Activity

In view of this potential for 'transition shock', how are student nurses and those who are meant to support them prepared for practice? You will find some answers in the next section. Find out in the Trust where you are undertaking practice placement experience what the policies and practices are in relation to helping the newly qualified nurse in practice.

Support for transition to being a qualified nurse

What has become known in the United Kingdom as the *Making a Difference* report (Department of Health 1999) and the subsequent later review of the 'fitness to practise' of student nurses, commissioned by the Nursing and Midwifery Council (NMC 2004), were both instigated by concerns from key health care stakeholders and the public regarding the skills deficit of newly qualified nurses. The recommendations from both documents included that students must experience a minimum of twelve weeks in their final clinical placement, which would include supervised clinical practice, with specified outcomes to be achieved for their entry to the register. This has been identified as a specific 'transition' period (Holland 1999).

One of the other key recommendations was that supervision be undertaken by an experienced mentor, who is charged with being a role model, a facilitator of learning, and an assessor within the clinical environment. To become registered mentors, practitioners must attend a 'preparation for mentorship' course accredited by the NMC, which requires that they achieve the outcomes outlined in the *Standards to Support Learning and Assessment in Practice: NMC Standards for Mentors, Practice Teachers and Teachers*

(NMC 2006a, 2008b). In the final clinical placement, students are also allocated what is known as a 'sign-off mentor', who has met additional criteria for supervision and assessment, and is accountable for the final assessment of practice and entry to the register. This confirms that you have achieved the required proficiencies for entry to the professional register (see Hart 2010).

In preparation for your final placement, it is important that you reflect on what knowledge and skills you already possess in relation to decision making—in particular, in relation to the role expectations of a qualified nurse. For example, if, on qualifying as a nurse, you work within the National Health Service (NHS) during your preceptorship year, you may well be expected to complete a portfolio of evidence that meets what are known as the Knowledge and Skills Framework (KSF) competencies. These were introduced into the employment criteria for NHS staff when, in 2004, the government at the time introduced its *Agenda for Change* (AFC). This was a pay system involving all health care professionals, a key strand of which is the NHS KSF (Department of Health 2004).

The intention of this is to enable you to identify the knowledge and skills that you will require to undertake the role of a newly qualified nurse. The KSF is also a tool that can help to guide your future development and progression. There are thirty dimensions, six of which are core and relevant to every post within the NHS, and which comprise: communication; personal and people development; health, safety, and security; service improvement; quality; and equality and diversity. (See **<http://www.effectivepractitioner. nes.scot.nhs.uk/practitioners/clinical-decision-making/core-skills.aspx>** to access the full NHS KSF document, information about the six core dimensions, and guidance on how to use the KSF document and competencies.)

⊕ Exercise

What do you think is going to be expected of you as a newly qualified staff nurse? Look at **Figure 13.1** and begin to write down your thoughts about decision making in the context of each of the areas. Refer back to **Part 1** in terms of theoretical underpinning and **Part 2** for examples of how you can link the NMC Standards and competencies, an example being **Chapter 5** on professional values and accountability.

The NHS Education for Scotland: Effective Practice site is one excellent resource that you can use to help you to begin this thinking about what is expected of you as a newly qualified nurse, and on 'being an effective practitioner'. It includes an excellent introduction to clinical decision making, and links to specific tools and online resources to support your ongoing learning about the KSF (**<http://www.effectivepractitioner.nes.scot. nhs.uk/practitioners/ksf-and-pdp.aspx>**) and about clinical decision making (**<http:// www.effectivepractitioner.nes.scot.nhs.uk/practitioners/clinical-decision-making.aspx>**).

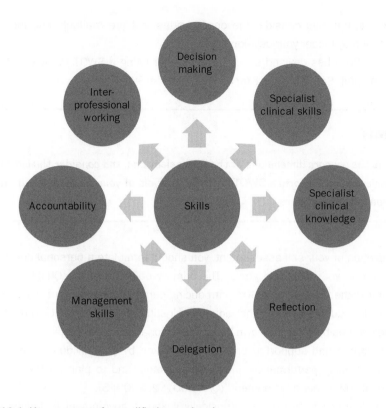

Figure 13.1 Key aspects of a qualified nurse's role.

Identifying personal and professional learning and development needs

In order to identify your learning and development needs, it is necessary for you to have an insight into 'self'. Warne and McAndrew (2009: 158) believe that 'preparedness' is linked not only to the technical and theoretical knowledge required for practice, but also to our attitude and emotions. Self-awareness is a challenging process that explores not only our learning needs, but also attitudes and emotions that are inextricably linked to our professional practice. According to Eckroth-Bucher (2010: 308), self-awareness is an intrapersonal process of self-discovery and that it is 'not a "thing" but instead a dynamic, introspective, interweaving, processing of thoughts, values, convictions, emotions, experience, and feedback'.

A self-assessment tool will help you to identify where you are now in terms of your decision-making skills, and will also highlight the knowledge and skills that you need to develop as a qualified nurse. One tool you may find useful is the SWOT, or SNOB, assessment tool, referring to **S**trengths, **W**eaknesses, **O**pportunities, and **T**hreats (SWOT), or **S**trengths, **N**eeds, **O**pportunities, and **B**arriers (SNOB), respectively. As you reflect on your current knowledge, skills, and competence, identify your strengths and weaknesses, but also consider the opportunities that are available and include any threats that may hinder your development.

Pearce (2007) has devised a ten step guide for using a SWOT framework that you may find helpful. See Table 13.1 for an example of a SWOT analysis.

Activity

Look at the six core dimensions of the KSF, select one, and consider the indicators for achievement. Perform a SWOT or SNOB analysis of your knowledge and skills in relation to the indicators.

On completion of your self-assessment, you should formulate a personal development plan based on your identified goals. The primary objective of the Quality Assurance Agency for Higher Education (2001) introducing personal development planning (PDP) is to provide students within higher education institutes an opportunity to reflect, plan and take responsibility for their own learning. Personal development planning is defined as 'A structured and supported process undertaken by an individual to reflect upon their own learning, performance and/or achievement and to plan for their personal, educational and career development' (QAA 2001: 2, 2009: 5).

Lifelong learning in the UK is intrinsically linked to government initiatives to support PDP for all health care professionals, in order that they develop the knowledge and skills required to deliver patient-centred care (Department of Health 2001, 2004, 2008). The NMC (2006b) reinforces the premise that lifelong learning is fundamental

Table 13.1 Example of a SWOT analysis in relation to the KSF core dimension 'communication'

Strengths	Weaknesses
Passed the communication OSCE in practice	Minimal experience of sharing decision making with others, including users of services
Received feedback from my mentors that I have good communication skills when talking to patients and relatives	Limited experience of the knowledge skills and attitude required for delegation
Motivated to learn	Lack of assertiveness
Able to recognize my limitations	Unfamiliar with the NMC guidelines and the legal aspects of delegation

Opportunities	Threats
Long final placement	Busy ward environment
Attend assertiveness training	Easily distracted
Review the literature, including the NMC guidelines and legislation on decision making and delegation skills	Poor time management
Practise delegation skills under the supervision of my mentor	Family commitments
Work with the inter-professional team	
Develop a personal development plan (PDP)	
Be supported and guided by my mentor	

to undertaking evidenced-based nursing within a complex and challenging profession. Personal development planning is a process of advancement and increasing self-awareness (Cotterell 2010), aimed at developing the knowledge and skills required for future development (Department of Health 2004). The benefits associated with PDP are increased confidence, independence, and problem-solving skills. The PDP cyclic process is a structured process that involves five steps, as follows.

1. Self-assessment
2. Planning
3. Doing
4. Reviewing
5. Recording

Each one of these stages involves decision making. The problem-solving approach of PDP will help you to self-assess your personal, academic, and professional development needs (See **Figures 13.2** and **13.3** for an example of a PDP and a completed PDP.)

In addition to and following your SWOT analysis, it is important to identify personal, professional, or academic goals, to which you should apply 'SMART 'criteria—that is:

- **S**pecific—goals should be precise and objective;
- **M**easurable—there must be a clear way in which to measure whether the goal has been achieved;
- **A**chievable—the goal must be achievable with available resources;
- **R**ealistic—the goal must be within your capability; and
- **T**imely—there must be a time frame allocated within which you are to achieve your goal.

Self-assessment	Goal	Resources	Criteria for success	Review date	Results of the review
I am aware that delegation is a skill I need to develop. I have little knowledge of what contributes to effective delegation, but I do have limited practical experience of delegation	To develop the knowledge, skills, and attitude required for successful delegation as a newly qualified nurse by the end of my final placement	Strategies for learning about delegation skills Observe health care practitioners on clinical placement Familiarize myself with the NMC Guidance on delegation Familiarize myself with legislation and Trust policies Identify opportunities to practise delegation within the clinical setting Source relevant literature and research articles			

Figure 13.2 Example of a PDP.

Self-assessment	Goal	Resources	Criteria for success	Review date	Results of the review
I am aware that delegation is a skill I need to develop. I have little knowledge of what contributes to effective delegation, but I do have limited practical experience of delegation	To develop the knowledge, skills, and attitude required for successful delegation as a newly qualified nurse by the end of my final placement	Strategies for learning about delegation skills Observe health care practitioners on clinical placement Familiarize myself with the NMC Guidance on delegation Familiarize myself with legislation and Trust policies Identify opportunities to practise delegation within the clinical setting Source relevant literature and research articles	Reflection observations Discuss with mentor to establish understanding Feedback from mentor Testimonial statements from other members of the health care team Practised delegation under supervision	02/02/2013	Reflection identified further developmental needs to improve assertiveness Positive comments from testimonial identified successful delegation

Figure 13.3 Example of a completed PDP.

Personal development planning will provide retrospective, current, and prospective evidence of your personal, educational, and professional achievements, providing the foundation for lifelong learning (Nixon 2008). Hibberd (2008) reiterates that self-awareness is an important component of lifelong learning: by understanding ourselves, we are able to understand others. Warne and McAndrew (2009) link this to the development of emotional intelligence.

Delegation and decision making

The forming of a personal therapeutic relationship is an essential element of nursing. The time constraints and stress experienced by nurses often encourage a task-based approach to practice, thus encroaching on the emotional and caring aspect of nursing. This may contribute to the development of a cynical and disillusioned view of nursing (Maben et al. 2006; Stacey and Hardy 2011). Effective delegation may help to free up nurses' time to enable the development of therapeutic nursing and the demonstration of greater emotional support—the effect, hopefully, being a more fulfilling experience of what it is to be a nurse.

More than ever, newly qualified nurses are expected to take on leadership much earlier in their careers than previously recognized (Young et al. 2004). Effective delegation skills are essential for leadership to succeed. Whilst some studies recognize a lack of student nurses' competence related to leadership (Wangensteen et al. 2008), confidence in student nurses' ability to delegate and to make decisions has improved since 1999 (Farrand et al. 2005). This is possibly the result of the implementation of the longer placements that students now experience following the implementation of a competency-based curriculum.

If you fail to delegate appropriately or efficiently, this will not only have a negative impact on patient care, but will also increase your stress levels. According to Maben et al. (2006), nursing workloads have intensified greatly over the last three decades, so delegation is a skill that nurses *must* learn. Reasons for these increasing workloads are many, and include the increased use of technology, faster patient turnover, and shorter patient stays. In their study of newly qualified nurses, Maben et al. (2006) found that having a lack of time contributed to nurses' stress and eroded their compassion, making them feel drained. Being able to delegate effectively can help you to combat some of this stress and help you to manage your time effectively. Not only can ineffective delegation be detrimental to you, but it can also demoralize your team. This may lead to impaired confidence among individual team members, but also in you as a leader (Weir-Hughes 2011).

Before you make a decision to delegate any task, you must ensure that care is appropriate, safe, and in the best interest of the patients (NMC 2008a). Many third-year student nurses find delegation a difficult skill to master and there are many reasons for this. Students in the final year of their programme are aware of the need to develop delegation skills, but feel that there are barriers that prevent them from doing so. Anecdotal evidence from students suggests that they often state 'I am just the student' and somehow do not feel worthy of asking a colleague to undertake a task on their behalf. Many students feel that they will be perceived as 'bossy' or as 'acting above their station', and so are apprehensive towards making decision to delegate tasks to other students, health care assistants (HCAs), or qualified nursing staff. Students feel the need to 'fit in' rather than to practise delegating to others. Often, there is an established culture within the clinical environment that can make it difficult to delegate to other members of the health care team. This overwhelming feeling of wanting to belong is often to the detriment of developing the skill of delegation (Duchsher 2009).

Effective delegation can be challenging for student nurses and newly qualified nurses. According to a study undertaken by Wangensteen et al. (2008), the key elements to successful delegation are for the nurse to have a good overview of the ward, to know the patients well, to understand the skills and limitations of co-workers, and to have confidence in themselves. However, confidence can take time to develop and involves continuous personal development, acquiring new knowledge, and learning through experience (Clark and Holmes 2007).

Exercise

Read the following advice offered by the NMC and the Royal College of Nursing (RCN) on delegation before considering **Case study 13.1**.

- <http://www.nmc-uk.org/Nurses-and-midwives/Advice-by-topic/A/Advice/Delegation/>
- <https://www.rcn.org.uk/development/health_care_support_workers/professional_issues/accountability_and_delegation_film>

The American National Council of State Boards of Nursing (1995) *Five Rights of Delegation* can easily be transferred to the UK health care setting, and espouses the NMC and RCN advice on delegation. The five rights can be used as a mental checklist for nurses when delegating tasks to others, comprising:

- right task;
- right circumstance;
- right person;
- right direction/communication; and
- right supervision/evaluation.

Use the NMC advice and apply the *Five Rights of Delegation* in considering **Case study 13.1**.

Case study 13.1 Leading and delegating

You are a newly qualified nurse working an early shift on a busy medical ward for the elderly. The shift started at 7.30 a.m. and it is now 8 a.m. You have just finished the patient handover and an HCA informs you that the senior sister is late for duty. Working alongside you is another newly qualified nurse, two experienced HCAs, and a third-year nursing student.

The consultant is coming to do her ward round at 8.30 a.m. and there is an inter-professional meeting that follows the ward round.

Questions

1. How will you coordinate patient care?
2. What are you going to do to prepare for the ward round?
3. How will you prepare for the inter-professional meeting that follows the ward round?

(Continued)

Case study 13.1 (Continued)

Issues to consider

When making these decisions about to whom to delegate tasks, you may want to consider the following from the NMC's *The Code: Standards for Conduct, Performance and Ethics for Nurses and Midwives* (NMC 2008a):

Delegate effectively

29 You must establish that anyone you delegate to is able to carry out your instructions.

30 You must confirm that the outcome of any delegated task meets the required standards.

31 You must make sure that everyone you are responsible for is supervised and supported.

Notwithstanding the NMC Code, there are some important critical factors that you need to consider when delegating, such as:

● your accountability—as the delegating nurse, you are accountable for the appropriateness of the delegation;

● your responsibility to patients and other members of the team; and

● appropriate risk assessment in line with clinical governance and supervision—you must ensure that an appropriate level of supervision and feedback is given to the delegate.

In responding to the questions, you need to decide who is going to coordinate the shift until the ward sister arrives. If you decide that it will be you, how will you delegate tasks or roles to the other members of staff on the ward? For example, your Band 5 (the grade attributed to first-level qualified nurses in the UK) staff nurse colleague could administer the medications to the patients on the ward. You are aware that the consultant is due to start her ward round. The third-year student nurse may offer to do the ward round as part of her learning goals, in which case you will need to ascertain the student's knowledge, experience, and understanding of both the patients, and their current health and well-being status, as well as the procedure of the ward round. (She has attended these before.) They could then prepare for the multidisciplinary team (MDT) meeting and give you a handover first. This will then leave you to prioritize care for all patients on ward.

You need to consider which skill you are delegating and to whom. You will have to clarify the skill or responsibility that you are delegating, taking into consideration advice on knowing the skills and limitations of the health care team (Wangensteen et al. 2008). For example, it may be that you ask the student nurse to undertake the ward round with the consultant. How will you check that the student nurse understands the role she is about to undertake? You may need to clarify each individual patient's need with the student nurse. You need to consider your Trust policy and the NMC Code (NMC 2008a) in order to guide you in deciding which tasks can be delegated to which member of staff. For example, there are certain tasks, such as administration of medicines, which can be undertaken only by a qualified member of staff.

Exercise

1. Consider how you can reduce stress around the issue of delegation.
2. Consider how you would aim to reduce stress around professional accountability.

Some of the possible responses to this action point can be found in the next section and throughout the rest of the chapter.

Accountability and decision making

'Accountability' is a word that worries many student nurses. It is generally recognized that accountability and responsibility are a major cause of stress and anxiety for both student and newly qualified nurses (Higgens et al. 2010). Being accountable involves knowledge, competence, confidence, and courage, and taking responsibility for your actions. However, in order to become confident and competent, it is important that you understand what 'accountability' means.

According to the RCN (2008: 6), accountability means 'being answerable for one's decisions and actions'. In order for you to be accountable for your actions, you need to be able to give a clear rationale for your care or omissions in care (Stanley and Eberhardie 2005). It is not acceptable, as a nurse, to perform a skill without having the underpinning knowledge (Roberts and Johnson 2009). As a qualified nurse, you are not only accountable to your regulatory body, but also to your employer and the general public (RCN 2008). One of the main ways in which you demonstrate this is through making a decision whether or not you wish to remain on the NMC register to be able to practise as a registered nurse. You are required to complete a 'notification of practice' form every three years, as well as to submit your annual retention fee payment. Failure to do so will result in your being unable to work as a registered nurse and could have other consequences in relation to your employment. See further information online at **<http://www.nmc-uk.org/Registration/Staying-on-the-register/Completing-your-notificat ion-of-practice-form/>**

It is important for you to remember that, as a qualified nurse, you have a legal, ethical, and professional sphere of duty for which you are accountable. You are also accountable for seeking support and advice, and for recognizing your limitations. Therefore you need to have an understanding of the legal, ethical, and professional factors in order to be accountable for the decisions that you make surrounding the care that you give. This can be when performing straightforward tasks, such as attending to a patient's hygiene needs, or performing complex tasks, such as inserting a urinary catheter.

Accountability involves making a decision and being responsible for the consequences of that decision. For example, you may understand how to undertake a wound dressing, but being accountable involves using the correct technique and best evidence to dress the wound, to interpret observations of how the wound is healing, and then to take appropriate action based on your observations. At the same time, you need to consider whether you have followed your employer's guidelines and completed the nursing documentation correctly. Similarly, you may be aware of a range of options to treat pain, but being accountable involves being able to choose the most appropriate method of pain relief based on your assessment of the patient and to offer a rationale as to why that was the best course of action. This type of decision making can be very daunting for a newly qualified nurse.

Autonomous decision making is defined by Beauchamp and Childress (2009) as self-rule, with the ability to exercise informed personal choice, and is fundamental in nursing. Becoming an autonomous practitioner may appear a daunting prospect, because it includes moral, legal, and ethical complexities.

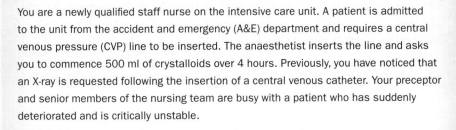

Case study 13.2 Following orders and challenging orders

You are a newly qualified staff nurse on the intensive care unit. A patient is admitted to the unit from the accident and emergency (A&E) department and requires a central venous pressure (CVP) line to be inserted. The anaesthetist inserts the line and asks you to commence 500 ml of crystalloids over 4 hours. Previously, you have noticed that an X-ray is requested following the insertion of a central venous catheter. Your preceptor and senior members of the nursing team are busy with a patient who has suddenly deteriorated and is critically unstable.

Questions

1. What factors are important when making your decision about whether to refuse to commence the infusion of fluids?
2. How you will communicate your decision?

Issues to consider

You are being asked to perform a procedure that you previously thought should not happen until an X-ray confirms the central line is in the correct position. You need to justify your reasons to the anaesthetist for not commencing the fluids and it is also important that your decision is based on clinical evidence and guidelines.

What are the ethical, legal, and professional guidelines that will inform your decision?

Case study 13.3 Making decisions when information may not be complete

As a newly qualified nurse, you are on the night shift and the nurse in charge asks you to complete the drug round for the patients, whilst she helps with an emergency admission. One of the children for whom you are caring has been admitted following a febrile convulsion and you notice that the paracetamol prescribed for 6 p.m. has not been signed for.

Questions

1. What actions do you take?
2. What factors are important when making your decision?
3. How will you communicate the information to other members of the health care team and the child's family?

Issues to consider

You need to inform the nurse in charge that the paracetamol has not been signed for and contact the medical team. You should continue to monitor the child's vital signs and inform the nurse in charge of any changes. You must document the omission on the drug prescription chart and in the care plan. You must also inform the child's parents and complete a critical incident form.

Overwhelmed and extremely vulnerable

It is natural for you to feel overwhelmed and extremely vulnerable prior to commencing your new role as a registered nurse. The transition process has been highlighted as potentially a stressful time (Deasy et al. 2010; Whitehead 2001). Towards the end of their course, students often vocalize feelings of uncertainty, insecurity, and trepidation.

During your final months of nurse education, there is often a realization that your role is going to change and the familiar will soon become unfamiliar. It is during this time that anxiety levels increase and you may begin to question whether you are prepared for your role as a registered nurse. Stress and anxiety expressed by newly qualified nurses is inextricably linked to accountability, responsibility, and decision making (Clark and Holmes 2007; Timmins and Kaliszer 2002). Students can experience a crisis of confidence that is often confused with a lack of competence.

An evaluation of pre-registration fitness to practise programmes in Scotland by Lauder et al. (2008) revealed that charge nurses found student nurses to be confident during their final placement, but subsequently lacking in confidence in their ability as a newly qualified nurse. The sudden reality of being accountable and responsible caused a crisis of confidence. Confidence is considered integral to learning and the anxieties experienced by students during their professional socialization into a new environment may inhibit that learning (Myrick and Yonge 2005; Roberts 2007). Feelings of anxiety and stress are not always perceived as negative, and there are times when stress has a positive effect, but ultimately it is how you cope with the stress that is important.

Reflecting on the day you commenced your nurse education, at times you may have felt overwhelmed and vulnerable—so what coping strategies did you find helpful? Stress management strategies should also be initiated at the outset of qualification as a preventive mechanism. At times, your transition may appear daunting and fill you with trepidation, but it is also an exciting time with immense opportunities. The impact of role transition on the newly qualified nurse may not evoke feelings of 'shock'. Gerrish (2000), in her follow-up study, found that although the transition remains stressful it was not as difficult as the nurses first anticipated. A key factor in the reduction of stress was attributed to nurses actively engaging in their own learning, supported by a programme of preceptorship (Gerrish 2000).

Preceptorship

As a newly qualified registrant (qualified nurse), these strategies will all help you to prepare for your role transition. According to Ross and Clifford (2002), newly qualified nurses who did not have a sufficient period of preceptorship (in other countries, this term is often used for pre-registration student support, whereas in the UK that is known as 'mentorship') found the transition traumatic. Your new post may be in an unfamiliar clinical environment and this may increase your anxiety as you start to form new relationships. A sense of belongingness within the clinical team is integral to your motivation for learning (Levett-Jones and Lathlean 2008); similarly, constructive feedback from a preceptor is essential (Deasy et al. 2010).

In 2006, the NMC provided *Preceptorship Guidelines* that strongly recommended a four-month period of preceptorship for newly qualified nurses (NMC 2006a). The NMC recognizes that the framework and time frame for preceptorship schemes is at the discretion of individual organizations. In line with the NMC, the Department of Health (2008: 52) published *A Quality Workforce*, identifying the need for a foundation period of preceptorship to help newly qualified nurses to begin the transition from novice to expert (Benner 1984) and to create the basis for lifelong learning. In 2010, a *Preceptorship*

Framework was introduced to provide guidance for NHS organizations in England providing preceptorship schemes (Department of Health 2010). The Department of Health defines 'preceptorship' as:

> *A period of structured transition for the newly registered practitioner during which he or she will be supported by a preceptor, to develop their confidence as an autonomous professional, refine skills, values and behaviours and to continue on their journey of lifelong learning.*
>
> (Department of Health 2010: 11)

The concept of assigning newly qualified nurses to an experienced nurse (preceptor) was intended to help the preceptee to develop further his or her clinical competence and confidence.

The responsibilities of a preceptor are identified by Myrick and Yonge (2005) as multifaceted, in that they are not only experienced practitioners, but also role models who guide, teach, and ultimately facilitate your professional socialization in practice. The role of a preceptor may appear similar to the role of a mentor, but you are now a registered nurse and professionally accountable for your actions. Accountability has been identified by newly qualified nurses as difficult because of their lack of experience and confidence in decision making (Whitehead 2001).

A preceptorship programme offers protected time for newly qualified nurses to access a structured framework that is aligned to their development, and which meets the aims and outcomes of organizational goals. The benefit of a structured preceptorship programme includes confident nurses, enhanced patient care, increased morale, job satisfaction, and improved recruitment and retention.

The Department of Health, in collaboration with NHS Scotland, has developed a website to support the transition from student to newly qualified health professional: <http://www.flyingstartengland.nhs.uk> One resource on the website maps the practitioner's progress in line with the six core dimensions of the NHS KSF. A newly qualified practitioner registered on the website will be able to access the ten learning modules. Completion of the learning modules will be evidence for your NHS KSF development review with your line manager. The online resources also include a section specifically for preceptors, with guidance and information on their role in supporting and facilitating newly qualified nurses. The preceptorship programme and your preceptor are there to help you through the transition, but equally preceptorship is an opportunity for you to identify your own learning needs. Identify the knowledge and skills that are relevant to your clinical area, but which are not presently included in your preceptorship programme. Formulate a PDP and discuss how you will achieve your goals with your preceptor.

Top Tips

A diary log is a useful tool that will help you to record your experiences. Your log will also help you to discuss with your preceptor the decisions you have made and to reflect on areas for further development.

As a newly qualified nurse, it is now your responsibility to take ownership of your personal and professional development: 'Lifelong learning requires an intention to learn, the development of self-awareness and the capacity to take responsibility for one's own learning' (Crick and Wilson 2005: 362). Continuing professional development (CPD) is a prerequisite for all registered nurses, and you will be required to complete a 'notification of practice' form confirming that you have met the post-registration education and practice (PREP) standards to maintain your professional registration (NMC 2011). PREP is a legal requirement that you must undertake to remain on the professional register and there are two separate standards. The CPD standard requires you to maintain a personal professional profile that may be requested by the NMC as part of its audit.

 Exercise

Obtain a copy of the *PREP Handbook*, available online at **<http://www.nmc-uk.org/Educators/Standards-for-education/The-Prep-handbook/>**

It features a template that you may find useful when structuring your profile.

As a newly qualified registrant, your CPD will encompass your development not only as a qualified nurse, but also as a teacher and facilitator of members of the health care team (Department of Health 2004; NMC 2008a).

Drawing on your experience as a student nurse, consider how, as a newly qualified registrant, you might address the issues identified in **Case study 13.4**.

Case study 13.4 Working with students

As part of your role as a newly qualified registrant, you are allocated to work alongside a registered mentor in supporting student nurses during their clinical placement. Tom, a student nurse on the mental health programme of study, is in his third-year second semester placement. Tom has been allocated to work with you on several occasions. Tom's midpoint interview is due, but the mentor informs you that she is on annual leave and asks you to facilitate the meeting. She also suggests that you raise

(Continued)

Case study 13.4 (Continued)

concerns with Tom regarding his poor attendance and attitude towards other members of the team.

Questions

1. What actions do you take?
2. How will you communicate your decision to the mentor?

Issues to consider

- What strategies are available within the clinical environment, Trust, or the university that will help you to inform and support your decision?
- What factors are important if you make a decision not to arrange Tom's midpoint interview?

Although you have worked with Tom on several occasions, your role as a registrant is to act as a role model and to facilitate his learning, but also provide feedback to his mentor. While it is important that you assess Tom on his progression, ultimately it is the registered mentor who is accountable for confirming that he has or has not met the NMC competencies (NMC 2008a). The mentor must arrange a meeting with Tom before she goes on leave to discuss any concerns and to develop an action plan that will enable Tom to address the issues raised. Once this has been agreed, you may then facilitate Tom's learning to achieve his identified goals. Reflecting on your own experience as a student nurse, you will be aware of the support mechanisms available to advise you when facilitating students to achieve their learning outcomes.

Throughout your career as a registered nurse, you could be asked at any time to demonstrate that you have continued to develop your knowledge and skills. A 'personal development record' and 'portfolio' are interchangeable terms that are used to describe a way of recording your CPD. Whichever system you adopt, whether paper record or e-portfolio, it must be an interrelated record of work-based learning, critical reflection (Timmins 2008), and a demonstration of your CPD.

The following top tips will help you to prepare for your transition from student nurse to newly qualified registrant.

⊖ Top tips

- Engage in PDP in order to develop your skills and knowledge.
- Never be scared to ask a question and never do anything you do not feel competent to do.

● Always have a rationale: if you do not know why you are doing something, always ask.

● Always be a preventative nurse.

....

Conclusion

This chapter has explored and discussed issues around decision making that may impact on your transition from third-year student nurse to newly qualified registrant, including delegation skills, challenging others, accountability, and prioritizing workload skills. These are only a few of the challenging areas which you will be faced with when making decisions as a newly qualified nurse. It has not been possible to consider scenarios that cover all of these and apply across all four fields of practice. The principles identified in the chapter can, however, be applied to similar decision-making opportunities. We hope that the chapter has helped you to plan your final placement as a student nurse and to identify specific developmental goals to facilitate your transition to registered nurse.

References

American National Council of State Boards of Nursing (1995) *Five Rights of Delegation: Concepts and Decision Making Process*, National Council Position Paper, Chicago, IL: NCSBN.

Beauchamp, T. L. and Childress, J. F. (2009) *Principles of Biomedical Ethics*, 6th edn, New York: Oxford University Press.

Benner, P. (1984) *From Novice to Expert: Excellence and Power in Clinical Nursing Practice*, Menlo Park, CA: Addison Wesley.

Bridges, W. (2003) *Managing Transitions: Making the Most of Change*, 2nd edn, London: Nicholas Brealey Publishing.

Bridges, W. (2004) *Transitions: Making Sense of Life's Changes*, rev'd 25th anniversary edn, Cambridge, MA: Da Capo Press.

Brown, M. and Olshansky, E. F. (1997) 'From limbo to legitimacy: a theoretical model of transition to the primary care nurse practitioner role', *Nursing Research*, 46(1): 46–51.

Clark, T. and Holmes, S. (2007) 'Fit for practice? An exploration of the development of newly qualified nurses using focus groups', *International Journal of Nursing Studies*, 44(7): 1210–20.

Cottrell, S. (2010) *Skills for Success: The Personal Development Planning Handbook*, 2nd edn, Basingstoke: Palgrave Macmillan.

Crick, R. D. and Wilson, K. (2005) 'Being a learner: a virtue for the 21st century', *British Journal of Educational Studies*, 53(3): 359–74.

Deasy, C., Doody, O., and Tuohy, D. (2010) 'An exploratory study of role transition from student to registered nurse (general, mental health and intellectual disability) in Ireland', *Nurse Education in Practice*, 11(2): 1–5.

Department of Health (1999) *Making a Difference: Strengthening the Nursing, Midwifery and Health Visiting Contribution to Health and Health Care*, London: Department of Health.

Department of Health (2001) *Working Together, Learning Together: A Framework for Lifelong Learning in the NHS*, London: Department of Health.

Department of Health (2004) *The NHS Knowledge and Skills Framework (NHS KSF) and the Development Review Process*, London: Department of Health.

Department of Health (2008) *A High Quality Workforce*, London: Department of Health.

Department of Health (2010) *Preceptorship Framework for Newly Registered Nurses, Midwives and Allied Health Professionals*, London: Department of Health.

Duchsher, J. E. B. (2009) 'Transition shock: the initial stage of role adaptation for newly graduated registered nurses', *Journal of Advanced Nursing*, 65(5): 1103–13.

Eckroth-Bucher, M. (2010) 'Self-awareness: a review and analysis of a basic nursing concept', *Advances in Nursing Science*, 33(4): 297–309.

Farrand, P., McMulla, M., Jowett, R., and Humphreys, A. (2005) 'Implementing competency recommendations into pre-registration nursing curricula: effects upon levels of confidence in clinical skills', *Nurse Education Today*, 26(2): 97–103.

Gerrish, K. (2000) 'Still fumbling along? A comparative study of the newly qualified nurse's perception of the transition from student to qualified nurse', *Journal of Advanced Nursing*, 32(2): 473–80.

Hart, S. (ed.) (2010) *Nursing Study and Placement Learning Skills*, Oxford: Oxford University Press.

Hibberd, P. (2008) 'Facilitating and assessment student learning: understanding the role of the portfolio', in K. Norman (ed.) *Portfolios in the Nursing Profession: Use in Assessment and Professional Development*, London: Quay Books, pp. 1–20.

Higgens, G., Spencer, R. L., and Kane, R. (2010) 'A systematic review of the experiences and perceptions of the newly qualified nurse in the United Kingdom', *Nurse Education Today*, 30: 499–508.

Holland, K. (1999) 'A journey to becoming: the student nurse in transition', *Journal of Advanced Nursing*, 29(1): 229–36.

Kralik, D., Visentin, K., and van Loon, A. (2006) 'Transition: a literature review', *Journal of Advanced Nursing*, 55(3): 320–9.

Kramer, M. (1974) *Reality Shock: Why Nurses Leave Nursing*, St Louis, MO: Mosby.

Lauder, W., Roxburgh, M., Holland, K., Johnson, M., Watson, R., Porter, M., Topping, K., and Behr, A. (2008) *Nursing and Midwifery in Scotland: Being Fit for Practice—The Report of the Evaluation of Fitness for Practice Pre-Registration Nursing and Midwifery Curricula Project*, Dundee: NHS Education for Scotland.

Levitt-Jones, T. and Lathlean, J. (2008) 'Belongingness: a prerequisite for nursing students' clinical learning', *Nurse Education Today*, 36: 103–11.

Maben, J., Latter, S., and Macleod Clark, J. (2006) 'The theory–practice gap: impact of professional–bureaucratic work conflict on newly qualified nurses', *Journal of Advanced Nursing*, 55(4): 465–77.

Meleis, A. I., Sawyer, L., Im, E., Schumacher, K., and Messias, D. (2000) 'Experiencing transitions: an emerging middle range theory', *Advances in Nursing Science*, 23(1): 12–28.

Myrick, F. and Yonge, O. (2005) *Nursing Preceptorship: Connecting Practice and Education*, Philadelphia, PA. Lippincott Williams and Wilkins.

Nixon, V. (2008) 'Assessment', in K. Norman (ed.) *Portfolios in the Nursing Profession: Use in Assessment and Professional Development*, London: Quay Books, pp. 21–46.

Nursing and Midwifery Council (2004) *Standards of Proficiency for Pre-registration Nursing Education*, London: NMC.

Nursing and Midwifery Council (2006a) *Standards to Support Learning and Assessment in Practice: NMC Standards for Mentors, Practice Teachers and Teachers*, London: NMC.

Nursing and Midwifery Council (2006b) *Preceptorship Guidelines*, NMC Circular 21/2006, London: NMC.

Nursing and Midwifery Council (2007) *Essential Skills Clusters*, NMC Circular 07(2007), Annexe 2, London: NMC.

Nursing and Midwifery Council (2008a) *The Code: Standards of Conduct, Performance and Ethics for Nurses and Midwives*, London: NMC.

Nursing and Midwifery Council (2008b) *Standards to Support Learning and Assessment in Practice: NMC Standards for Mentors, Practice Teachers and Teachers*, 2nd edn, London: NMC.

Nursing and Midwifery Council (2011) *The PREP Handbook*, London: NMC.

Pearce, C. (2007) 'Ten steps to carrying out a SWOT analysis', *Nursing Management*, 14(2): 25.

Quality Assurance Agency for Higher Education (2001) *Framework for Higher Education Qualifications in England, Wales and Northern Ireland*, Gloucester: QAA.

Quality Assurance Agency for Higher Education (2009) *Personal Development Planning: Guidance for Institutional Policy and Practice in Higher Education*, Gloucester: QAA.

Roberts, D. (2007) 'Learning in clinical practice: the importance of peers', *Nursing Standard*, 23(12): 35–41.

Roberts, D. and Johnson, M. (2009) 'Newly qualified nurses: competence confidence?', *Nurse Education Today*, 29(5): 467–8.

Ross, H. and Clifford, K. (2002) 'Research as a catalyst for change: the transition from student to registered nurse', *Journal of Clinical Nursing*, 11(4): 545–53.

Royal College of Nursing (2008) *Principles to Inform Decision Making: What Do I Need to Know Now?*, London: RCN.

Stacey, G. and Hardy, P. (2011) 'Challenging the shock of reality through digital storytelling', *Nurse Education in Practice*, 11(2): 159–64.

Stanley, R. and Eberhardie, C. (2005) 'Exploring the non-specialist neuroscience nurse's professional accountability', *British Journal of Neuroscience Nursing*, 1(2): 89–93.

Timmins, F. (2008) *Making Sense of Portfolios: A Guide for Nursing Students*, Maidenhead: Open University Press.

Timmins, F. and Kaliszer, M. (2002) 'Aspects of nurse education programmes that frequently cause stress to nursing students: fact-finding sample survey', *Nurse Education Today*, 22(3): 203–11.

United Kingdom Central Council for Nursing, Midwifery and Health Visiting (1999) *Fitness for Practice: Report of the UKCC Commission for Nursing and Midwifery Education*, London: UKCC.

Wangensteen, S., Johansson, I. S., and Nordstrom, G. (2008) 'The first year as a graduate nurse: an experience of growth and development', *Journal of Clinical Nursing*, 17(14): 1877–85.

Warne, T. and McAndrew, S. (2008) 'Painting the landscape of emotionality: colouring in the emotional gaps between the theory and practice of mental health nursing', *International Journal of Mental Health Nursing*, 17(2): 108–15.

Warne, T. and McAndrew, S. (2009) 'Mirror, mirror: reflections on developing the emotionally intelligent practitioner', *Mental Health and Learning Disabilities Research and Practice*, 6(2): 157–67.

Weir-Hughes, D. (2011) 'How to delegate', *Nursing Times*, 22 June, available online at <http://www.nursingtimes.net/nursing-practice/clinical-zones/management/how-to-delegate/5031439.article>

Whitehead, J. (2001) 'Newly qualified staff nurses' perceptions of the role transition', *British Journal of Nursing*, 10(5): 330–9.

Young, J., Urden, L. D., Wellman, D. S., and Stoten, S. (2004) 'Management curriculum redesign: integrating customer expectations for new leaders', *Nurse Educator*, 29(1): 41–4.

Further Reading

Burton, R. and Ormrod, G. (2011) *Nursing: Transition to Professional Practice*, Oxford: Oxford University Press.

Duchsher, J. E. B. (2009) 'Transition shock: the initial stage of role adaptation for newly graduated registered nurses', *Journal of Advanced Nursing*, 65(5): 1103–13.

Useful Links and Resources

<http://www.nmc-uk.org/Nurses-and-midwives/Advice-by-topic/A/Advice/Delegation/>

The NMC website provides specific advice regarding delegation.

<http://www.rcn.org.uk/development/health_care_support_workers/
professional_issues/accountability_and_delegation_film>

The Royal College of Nursing explores issues relating to working with health care support workers and delegation.

 <http://global.oup.com/uk/orc/nursing/burton/>

The Online Resource Centre for Burton and Ormrod (2011) offers some very useful resources, including some excellent podcasts by students on their transition periods and decision making. Listening to them will help you to think about your own concerns and excitement about becoming a qualified nurse.

Index